HEALING AND HYPNOSIS

ALSO BY WILLIAM SONG

On DVD
Self-Hypnosis 101

On CD
Brush and Floss Easily
Clarity of Mind
Healing and Surgery

HEALING AND HYPNOSIS

SELF-HYPNOSIS FOR HEALTH ISSUES

OR

A COMPLEMENTARY AND ALTERNATIVE MEDICINE APPROACH FOR PAIN, WEIGHT LOSS, TO STOP SMOKING, ETC.

WILLIAM SONG
CERTIFIED HYPNOTHERAPIST

HABIT PROJECT, SAN FRANCISCO, CA

Healing and Hypnosis

Published by Habit Project, San Francisco, CA
www.HProjectMedia.com

ISBN-13: 978-0-9767165-2-5

Library of Congress Control Number: 2008909447

Library of Congress subject headings:
Health
Self-Help
Self-Hypnosis
Hypnotism

Note on the font
For those curious about the font, it's Georgia (12-point). It's wider than the more common Times New Roman, so it's easier on the eyes. One interesting aspect of Georgia is its unusual look for numerals (see the ISBN above).

1.0

ABOUT THE AUTHOR

William Song is a certified hypnotherapist and NLP Master Practitioner. NLP stands for Neuro-Linguistic Programming; for simplicity, consider it a cousin of hypnotherapy.

He specializes in helping people with habits as well as those with chronic health conditions, including allergies, pain, and other issues that don't respond well to medication.

Years ago William suffered from chronic pain but made a full recovery, partly through harnessing the power of his subconscious mind. One of his goals is to show that chronic conditions can sometimes be temporary if the right tools are used.

He has a private practice in San Francisco, California. For more information, visit him on the Internet.

www.HealingAndHypnosis.com

DEDICATION

I dedicate this book to the many people suffering from health conditions who are frustrated by slow progress or who have lost hope.

If you've been diagnosed with a condition that's considered impossible to change, I'm here to say clearly, and loudly, that the word *impossible* is often in the eye of the beholder.

May this book help you to see your mind and body as more magnificent and powerful than you may have imagined. And may this book help you heal more quickly than you ever expected.

ACKNOWLEDGMENTS

Thank you to those who worked on this book.
- John Harrison, my editor. Your excellent advice made this book much better than it would've been.
- Kim Poole, my proofreader. Your sharp eyes saved me from major grammatical and spelling embarrassment!
- Marianne Smith, my friend. Your early draft comments helped me to simplify this book dramatically.

Thank you to those I've not met but who have influenced me.
- Richard Bandler and John Grinder, for developing Neuro-Linguistic Programming.
- Anthony Robbins, whose *Personal Power 2* audio program changed my life.

Thank you to my many teachers.
- Randal Churchill, Marlene Mulder, and the late Ormond McGill at Hypnotherapy Training Institute.
- Tim Hallbom, Kris Hallbom, and Nick LeForce at The NLP & Coaching Institute of California.
- L. Michael Hall, whose NLP writing workshop helped me to finish my book.
- My many clients over the years. I've learned so much from all of you.

"Give a man a fish, and he'll eat for a day. Teach him how to fish, and you feed him for a lifetime."

Chinese proverb

This book will help teach you how to fish.

TABLE OF CONTENTS

vii

INTRODUCTION:
CHRONIC PAIN COULD'VE
ENDED MY CAREER

Back in 1999, I began suffering from chronic pain. My arms ached, and some days I could barely work at my computer; my career in the financial field looked bleak. Without arms, how would I get my work done? Heck, how would I live?

One doctor told me that I'd be on pain pills for the rest of my life. But I refused to accept his opinion. He didn't understand chronic pain, and he sure didn't know my powerful desire to heal. I knew that I'd find a way to heal; I didn't know how I would, but I had faith I would.

Well, I found a way, and I'll say more on that later. After healing, I left my lucrative career in the financial field and found my calling as a hypnotherapist helping people to heal.

Let me be clear that I'm not healing people; clients do their own healing. The human body can be helped by surgery, medicine, hypnosis, etc. But it's the body that heals itself as much as it allows. I encourage you to view hypnosis as complementary to your healthcare professionals, not as a replacement.

In a nutshell, here's what you'll learn from this book.
- Basic hypnosis concepts
- Simple self-hypnosis techniques to help you heal
- How to write a hypnosis script to achieve your healing goal

By the way, using self-hypnosis does more than accelerate healing. Though this book focuses on healing, you can use hypnosis to reach goals in other life areas. Ready to start your adventure? Then let's go to part one.

Caution!
Hypnosis is a tool, not a miracle method.

This book is not intended as a substitute for medical treatment. Hypnosis can supplement the work you're already doing with your healthcare professional. The first step is to receive a diagnosis from your healthcare professional. After that, then consider using hypnosis as a part of your healing program.

Because hypnosis can be a powerful tool, throughout the book I mention areas to be careful of when using hypnosis. Read those cautions carefully to make sure that you're using hypnosis safely.

Nothing is 100% safe, but hypnosis, when used properly, is one of the safest tools available to accelerate healing.

Please consult your healthcare professional if you're going to use hypnosis by yourself on a health condition. It's good to keep them informed, and in some cases they can help prevent a potential problem that you may not have seen.

If you're going to use hypnosis on a serious or life-threatening condition, seek help from your healthcare professional and a hypnotherapist. Don't simply use a hypnosis book if the condition is that serious!

Why? Because an introductory book can't cover all the nuances of hypnosis. And sometimes nuances make a big difference. It's your health, so protect yourself with all the help you can get.

PART 1
HYPNOSIS SNAPSHOT

In part one, we'll cover the basics.
- Ch 1: Hypnosis Basics
- Ch 2: Myths of Hypnosis
- Ch 3: How Does Hypnosis Work?
- Ch 4: My Personal Healing Stories

Consider a different way of reading this book.
Instead of reading page-by-page, consider using a tip from speed readers, which is *to skim* rather than *read*. For example, you might look at the table of contents to get a quick sense of the major topics.

Then before reading a chapter, you'd look mainly at the headings and subheadings (in this book, that's mainly the bolded lines). Does it seem strange to ignore 95% of the words on the page? Well, skimming builds a mental framework.

Here's an analogy. You build a bookcase, but you have no books. Then you buy books, and it's quick and easy to shelve them since you already have a bookcase. It's efficient.

But if you bought the books first, and didn't have a bookcase, then you'd have to build the bookcase on the spot to shelve them. It would take time to shelve the books; it's not efficient.

In the same way, skimming prepares your brain to shelve ideas. Then when you actually read in detail, it's easy for your brain to shelve the ideas somewhere.

Bottom line: skim the entire book the first time you read it. Hold off on using the techniques until you're ready to read the book in greater detail.

"Knowledge of what is possible is the beginning of happiness."

George Santayana
Philosopher, poet

CH 1: HYPNOSIS BASICS

In this chapter, we'll answer these questions.
- "What is hypnosis?"
- "Why has hypnosis been such a well-kept secret?"
- "Is a stage hypnotist the same as a hypnotherapist?"
- "How does hypnosis work?"

Self-hypnosis compared to hypnosis

"Self-hypnosis" often refers to the hypnosis you do alone. But it's often said that all hypnosis is self-hypnosis, because in a sense, no one can hypnotize you. You're the one who enters hypnosis.

So for the purposes of this book, when I use the term "hypnosis," usually you could substitute the term "self-hypnosis." And if I talk about someone hypnotizing someone else, remember that even that is actually a form of self-hypnosis.

"WHAT IS HYPNOSIS?"

Depending upon who you ask, you'll hear many answers to this question. To keep this book simple, I define hypnosis in two words: relaxed focus.

Hypnosis is a natural state of relaxation and focus we experience each day. Here are a few examples of hypnosis.
- You daydream, meditate, pray, or do yoga.
- Time flies during a fascinating conversation.
- You intend to read a book for fifteen minutes, but an hour passes.
- You forget the last few miles you just drove.

Leonardo da Vinci, Albert Einstein, and Andrew Carnegie all used hypnosis. They focused their attention so effectively that they harnessed the power of the mind to solve problems.

Andrew Carnegie, the wealthiest American of his time (equivalent to Bill Gates today), hired Napoleon Hill to write a book called *Think and Grow Rich*. It's been a best seller for decades, helping many become wealthy. Yet it's a hypnosis book in disguise, teaching how to focus the mind.

"WHY HAS HYPNOSIS BEEN SUCH A WELL-KEPT SECRET?"

Well, no one group has tried to keep it a secret (though it may seem that way to some). Here are three reasons hypnosis has been misunderstood.

#1: Fear of the unknown.

Hollywood portrays hypnosis as mystical, magical, and frightening. But those who learn it find that it's natural, beneficial, and something we do under other names (i.e., meditate, daydream). They realize it's a tool, not anything magical.

#2: The hypnotherapy community lacks unity.

Many professions have a central body (i.e., the American Medical Association for doctors). It gives cohesion and a single voice. But my profession has no central body, no standardized training, no coordinated public relations effort, etc.

#3: The medical culture's been slow to adapt.

The American Medical Association approved the use of hypnosis in 1958, yet most doctors haven't been trained in it. But the medical culture is shifting, and I see two reasons.

A. Research shows hypnosis helps with medical conditions.

Hypnosis is one of the most effective tools in treating IBS (irritable bowel syndrome). Research shows that hypnosis helps with asthma, post-surgery recovery, chronic pain, and many health issues. Open-minded doctors have become curious.

B. Pop culture influences medical culture.

When the public sees celebrities such as Ellen DeGeneres and Matt Damon quit smoking through hypnosis, they ask their doctors about it. And then their doctors become intrigued about hypnosis.

"IS A STAGE HYPNOTIST THE SAME AS A HYPNOTHERAPIST?"

They're two very different professions.

A stage hypnotist entertains people.

He has audience volunteers bark like a dog, cluck like a chicken, and do silly things. To add drama, he creates the illusion of having great power over the volunteers. He hypnotizes volunteers to entertain the audience, not for therapeutic purposes. It's a show.

A hypnotherapist helps a client overcome a challenge.

It might be smoking, losing weight, or relieving pain. It could be a personal issue such as being more self-confident. Or it could be a business issue, such as overcoming procrastination, working more efficiently, or being a better public speaker.

Is there any overlap between these two professions?

Some stage hypnotists have a private hypnotherapy practice, attracting clients through their stage shows. He'll clearly explain to clients that the stage show is only entertainment, and private sessions are used to overcome an issue, and that the two are separate.

This distinction is crucial to make sure that the client understands that what they saw on stage isn't what happens inside the hypnotherapy office. The show is entertainment. What happens at the hypnotherapy office is not entertainment; it's for solving problems. I'll say more about this later.

"HOW DOES HYPNOSIS WORK?"

You have a lot of power inside your subconscious mind. This power can help you change beliefs and habits that hold you back.

Well, sometimes the body heals slowly, because it's hindered by a belief or habit. I realize that sounds strange, but a belief or habit can affect the body.

And if that belief or habit slows down healing, then hypnosis can help change the belief or habit, and that means you can resolve the block, thus getting the healing back on track.

For example, drug companies wanting to test a new drug will give the real drug to one group and a placebo (i.e., fake pill) to a second group.

Some who take a placebo during the clinical trial end up healing very quickly. Why? Because their subconscious mind's power is being tapped.

Bottom line: hypnosis can accelerate your body's natural healing process. Hypnosis helps you access power you already possess.

I'll say a lot more about how hypnosis works shortly.

CHAPTER REVIEW

"What is hypnosis?"
Hypnosis is a natural state of relaxation and focus we experience each day. It's relaxed focus.

"Why has hypnosis been such a well-kept secret?"
Well, no one group has tried to keep it a secret (though it may seem that way to some). Here are three reasons hypnosis has been misunderstood.
1. Fear of the unknown.
2. The hypnotherapy community lacks unity.
3. The medical culture's been slow to adapt.

"Is a stage hypnotist the same as a hypnotherapist?"
They're two very different professions. A stage hypnotist entertains people, while a hypnotherapist helps a client overcome a challenge. Some stage hypnotists work as hypnotherapists.

"How does hypnosis work?"
You have a lot of power inside your subconscious mind. This power can help you change beliefs and habits that hold you back. I'll say a lot more about how hypnosis works shortly.

- -

Next we'll talk about the myths of hypnosis.

CH 2: MYTHS OF HYPNOSIS

There are so many myths and misconceptions about hypnosis! Hollywood has made hypnosis seem mystical, magical, and frightening. The truth is a bit more boring: hypnosis is a normal part of life.

Hypnosis helps motivated people succeed, and it helps motivate people who want to be motivated. It's a tool, not a magic wand. When I give presentations, people often ask similar questions.

We'll look at some of those popular questions.
- "Am I asleep during hypnosis?"
- "Can I stay stuck in hypnosis?"
- "Will I forget what happened during hypnosis?"
- "Do people really cluck like chickens during those hypnosis stage shows?"
- "Is there any danger to using hypnosis?"
- "Can someone control me during hypnosis?"

"AM I ASLEEP DURING HYPNOSIS?"

No. You're in a state of mind between full consciousness and sleep. You can hear sounds, speak, move around, etc. Though you can experience the external world, usually you'd ignore it and focus inward instead. But if a fire alarm went off, you'd get up and quickly exit the building.

Cycling through Europe while in hypnosis

My client was going on a group bike tour of Europe. He was concerned about performing at his best, so I taught him a simple form of self-hypnosis. It helped him focus while being physically active instead of the typical self-hypnosis that requires relaxing and doing nothing else.

As he rode through Europe on steep and strenuous roads, he would hypnotize himself as he pedaled, and he outperformed what he'd thought possible.

When athletes talk of being "in the zone," they mean being focused yet relaxed, while performing at a high level. Remember the definition of hypnosis is relaxed focus! When athletes are in the zone, they're in hypnosis!

"CAN I STAY STUCK IN HYPNOSIS?"

Ah, Hollywood loves this myth, because it's so dramatic! But it's not true. In a hypnosis stage show, occasionally a stage hypnotist can't bring the volunteer out of hypnosis. Or occasionally during a session, a hypnotherapist can't bring the client out of hypnosis.

But the person isn't actually stuck in hypnosis. A small percentage of people go very deeply into hypnosis and experience tremendous bliss. They feel so good that they choose to stay in that blissful state. But they're not stuck; they're just enjoying it. They'll come out when ready, or if someone gives a compelling reason to come out soon.

"WILL I FORGET WHAT HAPPENED DURING HYPNOSIS?"
If you're at a stage show, the stage hypnotist may ask you to forget part of your experience. You might agree to his request or you might not. Or you might agree for a short time and then decide to remember what happened.

If you're seeing a hypnotherapist or doing self-hypnosis, usually you'll remember what happened. But a small percentage who go really deeply may not remember. Over the past few years of seeing many types of clients, I'd say that only about 5% have trouble remembering the session.

"DO PEOPLE REALLY CLUCK LIKE CHICKENS DURING THOSE HYPNOSIS STAGE SHOWS?"

Yes, volunteers cluck like chickens and act silly, because they trust the stage hypnotist. But they're not zombies. They keep their moral compass. Here's a popular stage show routine. The stage hypnotist tells the volunteer that the number seven doesn't exist for her. He asks her to count her fingers.

She'll count, "1, 2, 3, 4, 5, 6, 8, 9, 10." Notice she skipped the number seven, because for her it didn't exist! But don't worry, soon she'll have the number back.

But that was a harmless suggestion. If he had said, "Throw rocks and hurt people in the audience," she would've refused! The stage hypnotist pretends to have power, but it's all just an illusion for the sake of entertainment.

Insider's story (from a famous stage hypnotist)
Stage hypnotist: "One night I was doing a show, and a volunteer went into deep hypnosis. The guy was so impressed, he hired me to help him quit smoking. He went deep into hypnosis on stage, but not in my office. Unfortunately, he didn't stop smoking."

To me, this story is classic! It shows that the stage hypnotist has no mind control power. On stage, he's an entertainer, but off stage, he's a hypnotherapist.

His client got the two roles mixed up, hoping to get magically cured. Could the client have quit smoking through hypnosis? Yes, if he had understood that he, the client, was in charge of his success, and that hypnosis was just a tool to help him, instead of a magic wand replacing his efforts and motivation.

"IS THERE ANY DANGER TO USING HYPNOSIS?"
In general, self-hypnosis is extremely safe.

To put this into perspective, let's look at aspirin.
Aspirin is a safe drug, but a small number are harmed by it. Yet doctors prescribe aspirin, because it's helped millions of people. Yes, a small risk exists with aspirin, but the vast majority gain relief. It's a matter of balancing benefit with risk.

Yet here's the irony . . .
Some fear hypnosis more than aspirin, even though hypnosis is safer than aspirin! They fear the unknown; they've been hypnotized by Hollywood to believe the myths surrounding hypnosis! Those who understand hypnosis (i.e., medical professionals, researchers, etc.) find hypnosis to be very safe, definitely safer than surgery or medication.

What about the exceptions?
A very small number experience a negative reaction, but a skilled hypnotherapist can quickly handle this and calm the person. With a person doing self-hypnosis, risk is very small.

What about those with severe mental illness?
Severe mental illness creates less predictable, and potentially harmful, results during hypnosis. If this client is going to be hypnotized, it needs to be done by a hypnotherapist that is highly trained under the approval of a psychotherapist.

Perspective: malpractice insurance and hypnosis
Insurance companies set premiums high enough to make a nice profit. They set rates based upon risk. Doctors pay high premiums, because it can be a high-risk profession. Hypnotherapists pay low premiums, because risk is low. In fact, hypnotherapists can often pay more for auto insurance than for malpractice insurance!

"CAN SOMEONE CONTROL ME DURING HYPNOSIS?"
Perhaps control is too strong a word; let's use the term "influence" instead. If you're a parent, you influence your child to be kind and responsible. You influence your manager to promote you by doing a good job and being professional.

Society, advertisers, and politicians influence us.
Only some ideas influence us. It's partly about the message, the messenger, the technique used, and one's readiness to receive the message. We have much control on what and whom we allow to influence us. We manage influence.

Now back to hypnosis. In hypnosis, you do accept suggestions easily, but not all of them! You keep your moral compass. Learning self-hypnosis gives you more control of yourself by gaining greater control of your thoughts and emotions.

Is there any truth to the mind control myth?
Yes. The U.S. government (among others) tried creating hypnotic assassins that would kill and then forget that they'd been hypnotized. It sounds like a movie, but it's an obscure part of U.S. history. The government failed to create these hypnotic assassins and concluded that it was very hard to make people do something they didn't want to do. Whew!

Besides government experiments, anything else?
There have been rare cases of hypnosis harming someone. But before anyone panics, remember that it's extremely rare and doesn't apply to most of us.

Hollywood made people believe that it's simple to control people through hypnosis. The truth is boring, because the only one you gain control over is yourself. If you want to fear something, fear highly charismatic people and advertisers, the true experts in mind control.

CHAPTER REVIEW

"Am I asleep during hypnosis?"
No. You're in a state of mind between full consciousness and sleep. You can hear sounds, speak, move around, etc.

"Can I stay stuck in hypnosis?"
No.

"Will I forget what happened during hypnosis?"
If you're seeing a hypnotherapist or doing self-hypnosis, usually you'll remember what happened.

"Do people really cluck like chickens during those hypnosis stage shows?"
Yes, but they're not zombies. They keep their moral compass.

"Is there any danger to using hypnosis?"
In general, self-hypnosis is extremely safe.

"Can someone control me during hypnosis?"
No. The truth is boring: the only one you gain control over is yourself. If you want to fear something, I'd fear highly charismatic people and advertisers, the true experts in mind control.

- -

Next we'll talk about how hypnosis works.

CH 3: HOW DOES HYPNOSIS WORK?

We've gone over the basics of hypnosis and the myths. Now let's meet "Elizabeth." She's struggling with her weight, and her journey will help answer the question of how hypnosis works.

In this chapter, we'll answer these questions.
- "In a nutshell, how does hypnosis work?"
- "What's the difference between the conscious mind and the subconscious mind?"
- "Why does Elizabeth find it tough to lose weight?"
- "How does she reach her subconscious?" (nightclub analogy)
- "After she reaches her subconscious, how does she change the habit?"
- "How does this apply to other health issues and healing?"

Note about subconscious parts
I'd like to introduce the concept of a subconscious part. Let me be clear that I'm not talking about split personalities. The term *part* is in the context of a mentally healthy person who has different aspects of who they are. That covers almost everyone.

Do *parts* actually exist? Well, I can't point to them in a room; they're not physical. But then again, you can't point to someone's personality, either. Parts are aspects of a personality. They're not outside of a person; they are part of a person. Some argue that parts don't exist; they're just a useful fiction. Either way, it's useful.

What I've observed is that you can speed up progress by speaking to the parts. For me, that's a good enough reason to use the parts model of hypnotherapy, whether or not parts exist.

"IN A NUTSHELL, HOW DOES HYPNOSIS WORK?"

You have a lot of power inside your subconscious mind. This power can help you achieve your goal more quickly and more easily.

For example, your subconscious can accelerate your body's natural healing process. By going into hypnosis, you can communicate with your subconscious, asking it to help you access the natural healing power you already possess.

Sometimes the body heals slowly, because it's hindered by a belief or habit. I realize that sounds strange, but a belief or habit can affect the body. If that belief or habit slows down healing, then hypnosis helps you resolve the block. (And even if there was no block in the first place, hypnosis can still help to accelerate healing.)

Here's a quick overview.
1. If you want to change your beliefs and habits, speak to the part of you in control of your beliefs and habits.
2. Which part is that? It's your subconscious mind.
3. How do you speak to your subconscious mind? Get into a very relaxed and focused state of mind, also known as hypnosis.
4. Why does hypnosis help? During that relaxed state, your subconscious mind will accept suggestions much more easily. Therefore, you can influence it, and that helps you change your beliefs and habits more easily.

By influencing your own subconscious mind, you can harness that natural healing process your body would normally experience. This chapter goes into the deeper details of how hypnosis works. Let's start with the difference between the conscious mind and subconscious mind.

"WHAT'S THE DIFFERENCE BETWEEN THE CONSCIOUS MIND AND THE SUBCONSCIOUS MIND?"

Imagine a coin. You can't have a coin without it having two sides. Neither side is independent; a coin requires both.

Well, you have one mind with two sides: conscious and subconscious. Neither the conscious nor subconscious are outside of you; they are you. Neither exists without the other. They're interdependent and very different from each other.

Snapshot: conscious mind
- Logical, analytical
- Makes many decisions based upon logic
- Will power comes from the conscious mind
- What a person normally considers her true self (but the conscious part is only a small percentage of a person)
- Used when first learning a new skill
- Responsible for a small amount of our thinking and acting

Snapshot: subconscious mind
- Emotional, creative, impulsive
- Makes many decisions based upon emotion
- Emotional power comes from the subconscious mind
- What a person considers her intuitive side
- Stores habits and beliefs
- Controls most bodily functions, such as heart rate, breathing, and reflexes; it pretty much runs the body
- Responsible for most of our thinking and acting; basically runs your personality and much of your life

Internal conflict = subconscious mind wins . . .
When we have an unwanted behavior or habit, often this comes from an internal conflict between the conscious and subconscious. During that conflict, the subconscious usually wins in the long run.

That's why a person on a diet who's conflicted about it soon returns to overeating. Her healthy part may win, but it's only for a brief time. Soon the more powerful subconscious part starts overeating. To make this more concrete, let's meet Elizabeth, who's having a tough time losing weight.

"WHY DOES ELIZABETH FIND IT TOUGH TO LOSE WEIGHT?"

Each time she diets, she gains back the weight. Elizabeth thinks, "I'm highly disciplined and successful in all other areas of my life. So why can't I master my body?"

It's tough to stay slim if there's an internal conflict!
She doesn't know it, but she has a war raging inside.

- Her conscious mind, "Healthy Liz," cares about Elizabeth's physical and mental health. She makes short-term sacrifices for long-term gain. Figuratively, Healthy Liz is only five feet tall, skinny, and weak.
- Her subconscious part, "Party Liz," cares about Elizabeth's instant gratification. She cares only for today, for tomorrow may never come. Figuratively, she's ten feet tall, muscular, and strong.

Figuratively speaking, Party Liz is just really strong!
Healthy Liz and Party Liz aren't physical beings. They are aspects of Elizabeth. Party Liz isn't a separate person; she's a part of Elizabeth, just as being a woman is part of Elizabeth.

Elizabeth tried using will power to shed the pounds. But that didn't work, because will power is a tool of the conscious mind. And the conscious mind has little power over the subconscious mind. Party Liz is too strong, about twice the size of Healthy Liz. And Healthy Liz needs help!

Elizabeth needs to resolve this conflict.
What can Elizabeth do if Party Liz dominates Healthy Liz? Elizabeth needs to stop the fighting and resolve this in a peaceful way. She needs to convince Party Liz that good health trumps living only for the purely physical moment.

Since Party Liz is in the subconscious, Elizabeth needs to visit the subconscious. How does Elizabeth do this? Hmm . . . this reminds me of the nightclub analogy.

"HOW DOES SHE REACH HER SUBCONSCIOUS?" (NIGHTCLUB ANALOGY)

Let's use the nightclub analogy; let the disco ball drop!

A big bouncer's keeping people out of the club.

Elizabeth is not on the list, so he won't let her pass. Here's what she tried doing to get past the bouncer.

- Elizabeth used pure logic to convince him.
- Elizabeth threatened him.
- Elizabeth tried brute force to push past him.

How does she get past the bouncer who won't listen to logic?

Well, she's persistent and creative. She sees a very pretty female friend nearby and asks for a favor. The friend agrees, flirts with the bouncer, and Elizabeth slips past.

The nightclub is like the subconscious. The bouncer is like a filter blocking ideas from entering your subconscious.

Before Elizabeth used hypnosis, she tried talking to herself logically saying, "Exercise, moderate eating, and good health are great! There are so many benefits . . ."

But her filter blocked out her logical ideas. How can she get past the filter (i.e., the bouncer) so she can get her ideas into her subconscious mind (i.e., the nightclub)?

Hypnosis gets her past the filter (i.e., bouncer)!

By relaxing deeply, Elizabeth goes into hypnosis. In hypnosis, her filter also relaxes, allowing ideas to enter. In other words, she distracted the bouncer! And ideas get into the nightclub!

"AFTER SHE REACHES HER SUBCONSCIOUS, HOW DOES SHE CHANGE THE HABIT?"

She enters the nightclub and finds Party Liz (her subconscious part) sitting on a comfortable sofa. Remember, this is all figuratively speaking, to make it easier to learn the concepts.

Elizabeth speaks respectfully to Party Liz.

Since Party Liz is a part of Elizabeth's own personality, Elizabeth needs to treat her part with respect. It would be a mistake to shout at the part and get upset. That leads to more conflict. Elizabeth wisely speaks to Party Liz with respect. (To simplify this story, Healthy Liz remains outside the nightclub as Elizabeth talks to Party Liz.)

Elizabeth expresses her strong desire to become healthier.

Rather than just talk about dry facts, Elizabeth speaks from her heart, with real emotion about shedding the pounds as well as compelling logic about having great health. Party Liz responds best to logic plus emotion, not logic alone.

What happens after Elizabeth expresses her true desire?

At first, Party Liz listens politely but doesn't change the behavior. After weeks of visiting each day, Elizabeth finally convinces Party Liz that good health matters!

The result? Now Elizabeth exercises, eats right, and becomes healthier without so much struggle! Setbacks are quick and fleeting, and Elizabeth feels good about her path. She knows that this time, she's fully united!

The main tool in this book is the hypnosis script.

By learning how to write your own script, you can speak to your subconscious mind, helping unite your mind for a common goal. The script harnesses your power.

"HOW DOES THIS APPLY TO OTHER HEALTH ISSUES AND HEALING?"

If someone has an allergy, chronic pain, or simply isn't healing quickly, those could all be considered habits or patterns.

Most people think hypnosis helps with habits such as smoking and overeating. But hypnosis also helps with many acute and chronic health conditions. If something affects the mind or body, hypnosis can be part of the solution.

As I've said, hypnosis is a tool, not a magic wand. It helps a person harness their own power, but hypnosis by itself is like any tool; its effectiveness depends upon how skillfully the tool is used.

For example, a hammer is a great tool, but it needs a person to wield it effectively. Hypnosis also needs a person to wield it effectively. As you learn self-hypnosis, you are learning how to wield this tool.

Remember that hypnosis doesn't replace your healthcare professional. It complements them. If you're considering hypnosis for a health condition, I strongly advise that you get a proper medical diagnosis first. It could save your life! In a little while, I'll tell the story of how I could've died to illustrate further.

CHAPTER REVIEW

"In a nutshell, how does hypnosis work?"
You have a lot of power inside your subconscious mind. Your subconscious can accelerate your body's healing. In hypnosis, you can influence your subconscious to do that.

"What's the difference between the conscious mind and the subconscious mind?"
The conscious is logical and runs a small amount of our thinking and acting. The subconscious is emotional and runs most of our thinking and acting; it runs much of our lives.

"Why does Elizabeth find it tough to lose weight?"
She has a war raging inside of her, preventing success. To resolve the conflict, she needs to reach her subconscious mind.

"How does she reach her subconscious?" (nightclub analogy)
Remember the nightclub analogy? Elizabeth needs to get past the bouncer. In real life, she needs to go into hypnosis.

"After she reaches her subconscious, how does she change the habit?"
Elizabeth speaks to Party Liz, using powerful emotion and compelling logic. Elizabeth helps Party Liz understand that the old habit needs to change and that good health matters!

"How does this apply to other health issues and healing?"
Most people think hypnosis helps with habits such as smoking and overeating. But hypnosis also helps with many acute and chronic health conditions. If something affects the mind or body, hypnosis can be part of the solution.

- -

Next I'll share some of my personal healing stories to put what we've talked about into a deeper perspective.

"I can feel guilty about the past, apprehensive about the future, but only in the present can I act. The ability to be in the present moment is a major component of mental wellness."

Abraham Maslow
Psychologist

CH 4: MY PERSONAL HEALING STORIES

In this chapter, I'll share two of my personal stories.
- How I could've died in 2003
- How I recovered from chronic pain

The first story briefly discusses healing, but the emphasis is actually on a risk of hypnosis. The second story discusses the PEM triangle approach to healing, addressing the challenge physically, emotionally, and mentally.

HOW I COULD'VE DIED IN 2003

My stomach hurt all day. My wife urged me to see a doctor, but I didn't listen. I made one smart decision: I didn't use hypnosis to reduce the pain, because I didn't know why I felt pain. Reducing pain without a diagnosis is dangerous.

The next day, I still felt pain and was getting concerned.

Finally I called my healthcare provider on the second night, and the nurse said come to the hospital now. We went, and I got a shock.

The doctor said I needed to get my appendix taken out.

Since I hadn't expected this, I asked if I could come back. He said it could burst at any time. I stayed and had the surgery.

This was my first surgery, so I was scared.

What if something went wrong? Could I die? Scary thoughts raced through my brain, and I said to myself, "Hey, this isn't useful! I need to relax; I need useful suggestions." Within minutes, I'd taught my wife to hypnotize me, and I also did self-hypnosis. I taught her, because I felt comforted hearing her voice give me soothing hypnotic suggestions.

Surgery went smoothly, but here's the interesting part.

When I woke up, I didn't need any pain medication, and that surprised my nurse. I was up and walking in record time, and was discharged from the hospital quickly. How did I recover so soon and with little pain? Hypnosis helped me heal.

Bottom line: get a diagnosis before using hypnosis.

If you have a health condition, especially pain, get a diagnosis. If I'd hypnotized myself without knowing the cause of my pain, my appendix could've burst. And if I was in a remote location, I would have died. Get a diagnosis. It could save your life.

HOW I RECOVERED FROM CHRONIC PAIN

In 1999, I worked at an investment bank in equity research. I began suffering from chronic pain in both my arms from too much computer work. My boss was sympathetic, but my administrative manager said if I couldn't use my arms, I'd have to go. That scared me! I didn't want to lose my job!

Going through the workers' compensation system convinced me that it wasn't equipped to heal me. They gave me a bit of physical therapy and drugs, but I knew this wouldn't heal me.

One doctor outside of the workers' compensation system said, "You'll have to take pain pills and live with pain for the rest of your life." I said to myself, "Oh yeah? I don't think so! I will find a way to heal myself."

Desperate, I went outside the mainstream medical world and researched chronic pain. My goal was to gain a full recovery. Not a partial recovery, but a full recovery!

I worked a lot on my emotional and mental states.
Since I understood that healing the body had a lot to do with my mind, I used my background in Neuro-Linguistic Programming (NLP) to manage my emotions and focus. For this book, think of NLP as a cousin of hypnotherapy; for the purposes of this book, I'll just lump it under hypnosis.

Looking back upon that dark period, it's clear that the emotional and mental work I did was just as crucial as the physical work. The biggest physical therapy help came from the book, *End Your Carpal Tunnel Pain without Surgery,* by Kate Montgomery. At the office and at home, I did a lot of physical therapy on myself. A lot!

Finally, my PEM healing triangle approach worked!
PEM=physical, emotional, and mental. Because I tackled my challenge physically, emotionally, and mentally, I healed

despite working a full-time job that required extensive computer work.

I'll admit there were days that I was tempted to resign, so I could devote all my energy to healing. But I had faith that I could heal and keep my job; plus I needed the paycheck.

One reason I healed was pure determination.
During those painful times, my stubbornness, or as I like to say, determination, paid off. To me, living in pain for the rest of my life was not an option. I was driven to succeed. In my gut, I knew that I'd search for a cure until I found it. I had made a decision that 100% recovery was the only option.

No ifs, ands, or buts. Success was my only option.

Yet I realize that not everyone suffering from chronic pain has the advantage that I had.
My background in NLP really helped me. If I hadn't harnessed the power of my subconscious, I'd be popping pain pills today.

If someone hasn't suffered from chronic pain, they may not appreciate that the emotional and mental aspects are just as important as the physical pain itself. Had I only focused on the physical side, without aligning myself to 100% recovery, perhaps things wouldn't have turned out so well.

If you're suffering from chronic pain, or any chronic condition, I want you to know something important.
Many have reduced or eliminated their pain by addressing all three sides: physical, emotional, and mental.

No one fully understands the healing power of the body. So don't let anyone limit your healing, because the human body is capable of more than we realize. In my opinion, no matter how dire the case, we need to be open to success. And we need to be determined to do everything in our power to succeed.

CHAPTER REVIEW

How I could've died in 2003
If you have a health issue, especially if it's pain, please get a diagnosis. It could save your life!

How I recovered from chronic pain
Use the PEM healing triangle approach. And don't let any person limit your healing, because the human body is capable of more than we realize.

- -

In part two, we'll look at a hypnosis cookbook chock full of recipes, but you won't need to go to the grocery store. All you'll need are the following . . .
- A spoonful of curiosity
- A dash of an open mind
- And a cup of willingness to feel silly as you experiment

"Do what you can, with what you have, where you are."

Theodore Roosevelt
U.S. President

PART 2
HYPNOSIS COOKBOOK

In part two, we'll cover a few hypnosis recipes and a sample hypnosis plan. Because it's all techniques, there won't be any chapter reviews.
- Ch 5: Self-Hypnosis Foundation
- Ch 6: Stress Reduction
- Ch 7: Talking to Your Subconscious

Hypnosis complements your healthcare professional.
It's crucial to get a medical diagnosis from your doctor or healthcare professional, because hypnosis is not a health diagnostic system. Hypnosis is used after a diagnosis, so it's a complementary tool. If you haven't read chapter four, I urge you to do so. It could save your life.

Here are health issues where hypnosis has helped people.
- Asthma and allergies
- Cancer
- Chronic pain
- High blood pressure
- Insomnia
- Pre-surgery anxiety
- Smoking
- Weight management

By the way, I mentioned in part one to skim this book instead of reading it in detail, at least on your first time reading this book; then when you read a second time, it'll be easier to understand. Well that's especially important with these techniques. Skim the techniques the first time and hold off on practicing them. On the second time through this book, you'll be able to absorb these techniques more easily, and then it will be time to start using them.

"If one were to conquer in battle a thousand times a thousand men, he who conquers himself is the greatest warrior."

From the *Dhammapada*
An ancient Buddhist anthology

CH 5: SELF-HYPNOSIS FOUNDATION

We'll cover a sample plan and then some techniques.
- Sample Hypnosis Plan
- Countdown Technique
- Journal Exercise
- Power Phrase (automatic hypnosis as you sleep)

These techniques will give you a good foundation to start with, and the Power Phrase is a great way to start healing.

Sometimes a client will say, "William, I did the _____ technique, but it didn't work." After asking a few questions, I'll often find that the person missed a step. Or they didn't do it consistently. So do be careful to follow the steps and to practice. Understanding a technique isn't the same as mastering it, so please be patient with yourself.

SAMPLE HYPNOSIS PLAN

If this is your first time reading this book, I recommend skipping this page and the next page for now. Why save this page and the next page for the second reading of this book? Because it'll make more sense after you've read the book once.

"THE PLAN SEEMS SLOW. CAN I GO FASTER?"
Yes; it's only a sample. Feel free to speed up the plan.

"HOW'D YOU COME UP WITH THE TIME ESTIMATES?"
From my experience, most people take about two minutes to do the Countdown Technique and two minutes to do the Journal Exercise. The Power Phrase doesn't have a time estimate, because you keep saying it until you fall asleep. For the script listening, I estimated ten minutes, though your time could vary.

"YOU ONLY TALK ABOUT FOUR TECHNIQUES IN THE PLAN. WHAT ABOUT ALL THE OTHERS?"
Remember that it's a sample plan. You may prefer other techniques, so your plan may be different. Not every problem needs a script. Many problems can be solved with just the Hypnotic Parts Technique.

To get started, I recommend this sample plan. Focus at first on the Countdown Technique. That technique will help you get the most out of the other techniques, so take your time to become skilled at it (i.e., you can relax easily).

As you become comfortable, feel free to experiment with a technique not mentioned in the sample plan. Keep your hypnosis schedule light; if you're tempted to do too many techniques all at once, that could be counterproductive.

It's not about effort. It's about letting go and allowing yourself to practice and learn. Sometimes, less is more.

SAMPLE PLAN

Week 1 (6 minutes/day)
Countdown Technique
- Count down from 10 each day.
- 2 times/day, 2 minutes each time=4 minutes/day; I recommend morning and afternoon/evening.

Journal Exercise
- 1 time/night, 2 minutes.
- Do right before bed.

Week 2 (11 minutes/day)
Countdown Technique
- Count down from 10, increasing by 1 each day (i.e., first day starts at 10; second day is 11; third is 12, etc.).
- 3 times/day, 3 minutes per average day=9 minutes/day; I recommend morning, afternoon, and evening.

Journal Exercise
- 1 time/night, 2 minutes.
- Do right before bed.

Power Phrase
- 1 time/night, time is not applicable.
- Do this as you fall asleep.

Week 3 (11 minutes/day for techniques + 10 minutes/day for script=21 minutes/day total)
- Continue with all 3 techniques from week 2.

Hypnosis Script
- 1 time/day, 10 minutes.
- I recommend listening in the morning if convenient. It's a good way to start the day. Avoid listening right before bed, because you might accidentally fall asleep, possibly decreasing the script's power.

COUNTDOWN TECHNIQUE

Purpose: To go into hypnosis. You relax and do nothing.

Notes: It doesn't directly help resolve issues; it's a foundation skill that helps you to use other techniques. It's good to do right before other techniques, since it puts you into hypnosis.

1. Count from 10 to 1, slowly.

- Say, "10 . . . deeper . . . relaxed . . ., 9 . . . deeper . . . relaxed . . ., 8 . . ." until you reach 1.
- As you exhale, say one word. For example, exhale as you say "10," and then inhale. Exhale as you say "deeper," and then inhale. Exhale as you say "relaxed," and then inhale.
- Breathe as if the air was effervescent, like the fizzy air above sparkling water. Breathe lightly and naturally.

2. Practice once/day or even more often.

Helpful tips

Say the words out loud for the first week, and then do it silently. This technique develops relaxation, which is crucial when speaking to your subconscious. If random thoughts flow by, notice them, and then get back to the counting.

Breathe and speak slowly (i.e., instead of saying "deeper," say "deeepppperrr"). Words will approximate the exhalation length. After you're comfortable with 10 to 1, add a number each day. So 11 to 1, then 12 to 1, etc.

Perhaps link the technique to an existing routine, so it's easier to remember to do it. If you do it right before breakfast, then it's easier to remember to do it. Without linking, you may forget it. Doing it in the morning starts the day nicely.

JOURNAL EXERCISE

Purpose: To record your progress, help focus your mind on appreciation, and help keep you on track.

Notes: This technique takes about two minutes.

1. Right before bed, get out your journal.

2. Jot down these things briefly.
- What hypnosis exercises you did that day
- Interesting thoughts or experiences related to your goal, and possibly even a thought outside of the goal

3. Jot down two appreciations about the day.
- Examples: The sun was shining. I have a roof over my head. An old friend called for the first time in years! I live in a great city. I have two eyes to read with.
- Having appreciation right before bed puts your mind into a positive frame, increasing your sleep quality. People who watch the news before bed can disturb their sleep.

Helpful tip

A traditional journal records your daily reflections, frustrations, and life experiences. If you keep a traditional journal, write in that one earlier. Keep this hypnosis journal totally separate. You don't want to mix the emotions of the traditional journal in with your ritual of writing in your hypnosis journal.

This is a foundation skill that's easy to underestimate. People who keep a hypnosis journal tend to succeed faster than the people who don't.

POWER PHRASE
(AUTOMATIC HYPNOSIS AS YOU SLEEP)

Purpose: Helps you achieve your goal as you sleep.

Notes: This is one of the most powerful techniques in this book. In structure, it's similar to the Countdown Technique. But this one directly helps you achieve your goal.

1. Think of a phrase that reflects what you want.

- State it in the positive. Say what you want rather than what you don't want. If you smoke, you'd say, "I want to be healthy, breathing easily." You wouldn't say, "I don't want to smoke." I'll say more about this in the script section.
- Experiment with the present tense and other tenses. For example, "I am healthy" versus "I am healthier each day." One tense may work better for you.
- The phrase needs to make you feel really good. A strong emotion is the key behind this technique! If that's absent, then refine the phrase.

2. Each night as you fall asleep, repeat the phrase as you count from 10 to 1.

- Say, "10 . . . [the phrase] . . ., 9 . . . [the phrase] . . ."
- You may fall asleep before reaching one, but if you're still awake, repeat the sequence until you fall asleep.
- Watch a movie of yourself on your mental movie screen as that person who's succeeded. You see yourself and deeply feel the emotions.

3. When you awaken in the morning, repeat just the phrase three times. Then open your eyes and get out of bed.

- To speed up progress, say the phrase throughout the day and play your movie with full emotion.

Client story

I remember an anxious client who made impressive progress. She used hypnosis to rapidly resolve multiple challenges. Family problem? Solved it. Career challenge? Solved it. Personal problem? Solved it.

Though I was impressed at her speed and skill, what really stood out was her quick mastery of the Power Phrase. Within days of using it, she resolved a major anxiety that had blocked her happiness for a long time. Not everyone masters this technique as quickly as she did, but I did want to show the potential power of this simple technique.

Helpful tips

It's crucial to practice for 30 nights minimum! More is even better. Missing a night can hinder progress. Momentum is a huge factor for this technique.

If you're not progressing, refine your phrase. Or even edit your movie. The phrase needs to resonate deeply with you, and the movie needs to resonate deeply with you. In short, strong emotion is key. Both the phrase and movie need to be powerful to get the most benefit from this technique.

Sample phrases

"I am healthy."
"Each day I become healthier."
"Each day my hip heals faster."
"Each day I shed four ounces of excess weight."
"My back feels better each day."
"My body feels better and better."
"Happiness is a choice, so I choose to be happier each day."

"Remember that happiness is a way of travel—not a destination."

Roy M. Goodman
American politician

CH 6: STRESS REDUCTION

In this chapter, we'll cover these techniques.
- 8:15 Solution
- 24 Hours Technique
- What if . . . You Were to Pass Away Technique
- What if . . . Someone Were to Pass Away Technique

Some believe that stress has more to do with life events, or their external world. They're happy during good times, but they're sad during tough times. Unfortunately, that makes happiness random, since life isn't 100% under their control.

To me, stress has more to do with focus, or the internal world. This means being happy during tough times and good times. I'm not saying that life events have no effect; what I'm saying is that focus influences how we experience those life events.

During high school, I fell apart. Wasn't sure I'd even graduate.
Before senior year, I was a pretty well-adjusted kid who got good grades and stayed out of trouble (usually). But in the latter part of high school, I spiraled downward into despair.

Without going into all the details, let's just say that I ran into classic teenage problems and didn't know how to deal with them. I'm not claiming that my problems were worse than what others go through. I just didn't deal with them very well.

My grades slipped badly, and I felt I might not graduate. Of course the danger of not graduating may have had to do with my skipping school often and not doing my homework.

But I just didn't care; I stopped caring about school, my future, and my life. When I peered into the future, I saw nothing. I don't mean that figuratively; I'm talking literally. It was as if someone had put a dark curtain over my eyes. I couldn't see beyond it.

I walked the streets at night, hoping to hurt someone. Since I didn't know how to deal with my problems, rage and raw emotion coursed through my veins. The emotions were so strong that I wanted to hurt someone, anyone, who looked at me in the wrong way. I needed to lash out.

Fortunately, the streets I walked were safe, and no one ever bothered me during my nightly walks. As I look back upon those dark times, I'm grateful that I didn't hurt anyone, and I'm grateful that I didn't get hurt! Maybe people sensed my anger and steered clear of me, or maybe it was just luck.

But despite the despair of youth, I did survive. Somehow, I climbed out of the pit. And after I climbed out, I felt I could see. The world looked so different!

Before, all I saw was darkness. Now that I was out of the pit, I saw light. I saw a future for myself. The dark curtain had been lifted, and it got replaced by profound lessons.

I learned that the past, no matter how painful it was for me, could be my resource rather than a burden. I could use my past to become stronger and learn from my mistakes. And I found that happiness is more internal than external, and though it comes with a high price, it is a choice. I chose happiness.

I used to think, "Happiness is for some people, but it's just not for me. I can't be that way." That's how I used to think, until I realized that happiness wasn't handed to people. I had to get it myself. And I found that for me, happiness was a process more than a destination. It became something I had to create inside, or allow myself to experience each day, not something that I had to wait for to enter my life.

How did I climb out of the pit? I don't know.
How did I realize that happiness was a choice? I'm not sure. If I had a step-by-step formula for how I went from despair to happiness, I'd share it. It's fuzzy as to how it all happened.

The entire process took me years, because I kept making mistakes along the way. Maybe "mistakes" isn't the correct word; how about I kept needing reminders.

Being a victim can be tough to give up.
I took great comfort in defining myself by my past or as a victim. I played that role long enough and enjoyed it on some perverse level. It wasn't easy to let go of that role, to let go of that rage, that entitlement. But I did break out of that mental prison and empathize with people who are still trapped.

Deep in my heart, I feel that every single one of us, no matter how hurt, how injured, has the power to become truly happy. I've seen many clients let go of the past and free themselves from their mental prisons, and in some cases, their newfound happiness helped create profound positive changes in their family members or friends. Happiness can be contagious!

Had I known about hypnosis back then, I could've avoided a lot of suffering. I learned the hard way, and I feel that we're not meant to suffer. We're meant to thrive.

What does this have to do with healing?
The mind and body are interdependent, affecting each other. Hypnosis isn't a cure-all. But it's a tool to be considered, especially when someone's done everything possible on the physical level. I've seen many clients resolve chronic health conditions by shifting their beliefs and habits.

Hypnosis doesn't always work, but it has helped many people. My goal isn't to convince everyone that my views are right. I've simply shared my experience, and it will resonate with some of those who hear this message.

8:15 SOLUTION

Purpose: To do all your worrying only once per day, so you can feel good the rest of the day.

Notes: "Worry" is endless-loop thinking that makes you feel bad and is unproductive. It's not the same as solution-oriented thinking, which is productive.

1. Set aside a time to do all your worrying. Let's use 8:15 PM as an example.
- Make a deal with yourself to only worry at 8:15 PM for a certain time period (such as fifteen minutes).
- If a worry pops up at another time, say, "Oh, it's not 8:15 yet. I'll jot it down for my 8:15 worry list."
- During the day, you may think about upsetting thoughts in a constructive way. For example, "What can I learn from the experience? How can I benefit from it? Would I do anything differently next time? Does that other person have some real issues?" But save worry thoughts for 8:15 PM.

2. At 8:15 PM, worry for your allotted time.
- Let yourself worry to your heart's content! Perhaps start off at fifteen minutes. Don't do any productive thinking during this time. If you have a useful thought, jot it down for after you're done worrying. Right now, useful thoughts aren't welcome; your only focus is to worry, worry, and worry. Force yourself to only worry! If that's tough, keep on forcing the worries!

3. When your time's up, you're done.
- You made a promise to yourself to only worry at 8:15 PM. Once your time's up, you're done. Now you're free to think of useful thoughts.

Unemployed and sinking fast!
Shortly after graduating from college, I moved to San Diego. One of my dreams was to become wealthy by having my own money management firm. But I needed a job to learn the ropes.

My job search went nowhere, so I worked briefly as a grocery store bagger and then at a minimum wage job at a Mexican restaurant. And I interned at a small money management firm (for free) that I knew had no interest in hiring anyone.

Months later, my self-esteem and optimism had faded. Frustration and depression snowballed. It wasn't as bad as my high school pit of despair, but I was worrying. My head felt like it would explode! On the bright side, I didn't want to lash out at the world.

In sheer desperation, I had a talk with myself. "This isn't healthy! Worrying all the time isn't going to get me a job. But what can I do but worry? Hey, what if I save my worry for a few minutes each night? Maybe that could work!"

Out of that conversation, the 8:15 Solution was born. And I transformed my worries into concern, and concern into action. Something positive came out of this tough time.

Helpful tip
As you repeat this exercise each day, you may notice something odd. Your subconscious may gradually realize that worry is unproductive. It realizes that thoughtful analysis is different from worry, and that worry is a waste of time and energy.

And soon, when 8:15 PM rolls around, you may find yourself thinking, "I'm not in the mood to worry." You're training yourself to realize that worry isn't useful. Then you'll dramatically reduce worrying or perhaps even eliminate it.

---

24 HOURS TECHNIQUE

Purpose: Reduce stress; put things into perspective.

Notes: Many find this exercise eye-opening, because they've never calculated their free time in this way.

Imagine driving home on Friday evening. Suddenly, a driver cuts into your lane, almost hitting you. As he speeds away, you get mad, thinking, "That idiot almost crashed into me!" Though you're with friends, you're mad the rest of the night.

How can you move past that incident? Put it into perspective.

1. Ask, "How do I use my 24 hours per day?"
- Approximate numbers and averages are fine.
- No one's grading your paper. Most will total up to about 21 hours or so. That leaves three hours for errands, time with friends/family, relaxation, etc. If you watch TV, that eats up a chunk of time.

2. Ask, "How much time is it worth to think about this stressful experience?"
- Take a moment to think that most of your time is spoken for, so how much free time do you really have?

3. Ask, "What can I learn from the experience?"
- If you had it to do over again, how could you have done things differently?
- How would you like to feel if this happens again?
- If you learn something from each experience, you've gained knowledge that can help you in the future. Often something can be learned.

Example with Kiefer, professional dog walker
Kiefer walks his dog clients across the street, when suddenly a cyclist zooms by, almost hitting his dogs. Upset, Kiefer yells at him. At the park, Kiefer uses this technique for the first time.

Kiefer's Step 1 (he uses averages and estimates)

8 hours	Sleeping (yes, he sleeps eight hours)
1 hour	Shower; eat breakfast; get ready for work
½ hour	Drive to dog owners to pick up dogs
9 hours	Walk dogs; eat lunch; do paperwork
½ hour	Drive to drop off dogs to owners
1 hour	Prepare dinner; eat dinner
1 hour	Wash dishes; tidy up home
21 hours	

He thinks, "I've got three hours a day? That's not much."

Kiefer's Step 2
He asks himself, "How much time is it worth to think about that cyclist? I have three hours a day. But he doesn't deserve my time or energy. I'll give him a few minutes, but that's it."

Kiefer's Step 3
After he finishes thinking about the cyclist for a few minutes, he asks himself, "What can I learn from this experience? I thought I was careful crossing, but that cyclist came so fast! He needs to slow down and be more careful!"

Then Kiefer thinks, "Maybe I can also look and listen even more carefully. If this happens again, how would I like to feel? I don't know, I hate to think my dogs could get hurt. If this happens again, I'd like to feel more calm afterwards."

Then he thinks, "What did I learn today? I really care about my dogs, and I want them safe. I get angry if they're threatened. And maybe, I can be a little more careful crossing the street with my dogs. But man, that cyclist was going too fast!"

Notes about Kiefer's three steps

Now and then he got caught up in anger at the cyclist, but for the most part, Kiefer did a good job with the technique. He'll do even better with practice, but for a first attempt, he did great. And soon, he may not need to use this technique.

Helpful tip

Do this with full emotion, with all your heart. Don't simply read it and go through the motions. Put yourself fully into it.

As you practice, you may find that fewer things bother you.

And that driver who cut you off isn't entitled to take more of your time or energy.

You're training your subconscious to put stressful events into perspective. It will realize, "Hey, my free time's limited each day. Do I want to spend it thinking about ____? Or would I rather enjoy my free time?" Then it will help you to choose to enjoy your free time.

WHAT IF . . . YOU WERE TO PASS AWAY TECHNIQUE

Purpose: Treat yourself with more kindness, respect, and understanding.

Notes: Some people may find this technique morbid. Some may find it liberating. Use it if you dare. This goes well with the next technique.

1. Ask yourself, "If I had an incurable condition that could kill me at any time without warning, how would I spend my life?"

2. Ask yourself, "And how would I interact with my loved ones and everyone else?"

3. Appreciate that you don't have an incurable condition, and that you do have time to live.
- If you actually do have an incurable condition, simply appreciate whatever time you have left. And by the way, sometimes *incurable* really means that the health professional doesn't know how to cure it. I've witnessed clients with incurable, or chronic, conditions heal themselves with hypnosis as part of their solution.

Example with George, a project coordinator of a baseball team
George and his girlfriend went out with his good friends Jerry and Elaine. Unfortunately, Elaine accidentally embarrassed George that night.

Elaine later apologized. In the past, George would've stewed over the incident for days or weeks. But instead of being so upset, George experimented with this technique. He asked himself, "If I had an incurable condition that could kill me at any time without warning, how would I spend my life?"

53

And he answered, "I'm not sure, but I'm pretty sure I wouldn't waste it thinking about embarrassing moments. Maybe I'd enjoy each day a bit more or do things I'd been putting off . . . You know, thinking about death is helping me realize that those small things, like what Elaine did last night, don't matter."

Then George ponders his job. "I don't like office politics, but there's always some office politics, even when people get along. But if I might die at any time, do I want to waste my time on office politics? No! I want to do my job, be friendly with people, and stay out of petty things. From now on, if someone starts gossiping, I won't gossip back. Yup, that's how I want to be."

Then George ponders his family. "What about my parents? Could I treat them better? I think I could be a better son."

By the way, this technique goes well with the next technique. They're kind of a package deal.

Helpful tip

This may help deepen this technique for you. The hypothetical question (i.e., incurable condition that could kill me at any time without warning) isn't hypothetical. I've had a terminal condition since birth, and this condition could kill me at any time without warning. But don't feel sorry for me, because I've learned to accept it and appreciate my blessings even more.

What's the name of my incurable condition? It has four letters. L-I-F-E. And you have the same condition that I do. You have a life, and I have a life, and neither of us knows when we'll die. All we control is what we do with the time we're given.

How much time do you want to spend on petty things?

WHAT IF . . . SOMEONE WERE TO PASS AWAY TECHNIQUE

Purpose: Treat a loved one (i.e., family member, friend, etc.) with more kindness, respect, and understanding.

Notes: Some people may find this technique morbid. Some may find it liberating. Use it if you dare. This goes well with the previous technique.

1. Ask yourself, "If so-and-so passed away today, would I have any regrets?"

2. List those regrets on paper or mentally.

3. Appreciate that they're still alive, and take action to prevent those regrets.

Here's a personal example of the technique.
I asked myself, "If my parents passed away, would I have any regrets?" Here are a few things from my list.
- I would regret not telling them that I love them a bit more often than I had.
- I would regret not visiting more often.
- I would regret not calling more often.
- I would regret not telling them that I appreciate the sacrifices they've made to raise me.
- I would regret not doing small things that would've made them happier.

When I was a young adult, it drove me crazy to hear my mom treat me like a kid when I visited. She'd say, "Make sure to dress warmly. You don't want to catch a cold." But after realizing the fragility of life, knowing that one day she wouldn't be around to tell me to dress warmly, I almost cried. Even as I'm writing this, I can feel tears welling up.

After I came up with the list of regrets, I took action to make things better. I visited my parents more, called more, etc. I strived to become a better son, and though I wasn't always successful at it, I made the effort more than I had before.

The past is over, and I can't undo hurtful things I've said or done. But I do control what I do today. This technique has helped me let go of petty things (okay, most petty things) and focus on what's real, such as appreciating positive things about my family. Thinking about death can help us treat people better while they're alive.

Helpful tips

Start small. If there's one small thing you can do, start there. As I mentioned, one small thing I did was to call my parents more often.

Instead of focusing on being the perfect son, I decided to be a better son than before. That decision was more realistic.

In my opinion, when we try to be perfect, we can get caught up by all our options and end up doing little. Letting go of perfection frees up our energy, makes us feel better, and allows us to act.

CH 7: TALKING TO YOUR SUBCONSCIOUS

In this chapter, we'll cover these techniques.
- Hypnotic Parts Technique
- Transform Your Inner Critic

It's tough to reach a goal when you feel conflicted. It's time to clear up conflicts by speaking to your subconscious mind. You may remember Elizabeth and the nightclub analogy (chapter three) as she spoke to Party Liz. We'll revisit Elizabeth soon, but first let's talk more about parts.

Parts are not split personalities. *Parts* are normal.

I talked about *parts* in chapter three, and I'll say more now. People with a split personality, severe disassociation issues, or other mental illness need to see a psychotherapist, because some forms of hypnosis can be dangerous for those people.

Fortunately, most of us are in good mental health. For us, we express internal conflict in a safer way, through our parts. Imagine you're home alone and see a plate of cookies. You might say, "Part of me wants a cookie, but maybe I shouldn't."

You understand that the part that wants the cookie isn't separate from you, but is an aspect of you, or a role you have. At home, you play the role of parent and spouse. At lunch with friends you play the role of friend. At work you play the role of manager or staff member. These roles aren't outside of you; they are aspects of you. They are parts of your identity.

Benefits of speaking to your subconscious parts
- Resolve some issues just by talking to your parts.
- Gain a sense of how to resolve issues, which helps you write a better hypnosis script.
- Strengthen the bond between the conscious and subconscious.
- Maintain a healthier balance in your life.
- Prevent problems from happening.

Let me explain that last point with the good friend analogy.
Imagine spending time with your good friend on a regular basis. You both understand what's on each other's mind.

You help each other out, deepening trust and the bond of friendship. You look out for each other, helping each other see things more clearly, even avoiding problems before they happen. Well, your subconscious can advise you on how to deal with small problems before they become big ones or even help avoid problems entirely!

It's kind of similar to someone who's physically fit.
If someone eats healthy food, exercises, and takes care of herself, she helps prevent illness, and she often gains more energy. This can then snowball into positive changes in other areas of life.

By you having a strong bond between your conscious and subconscious, you boost your power physically, emotionally, and mentally. Talking to yourself is something you've done naturally all your life, and now it's time to learn how to do it even more effectively.

And as you strengthen this skill, you'll become healthier and reach other goals faster and more easily. You're building a stronger bond to yourself, and that relationship is one of the best ones you could have.

HYPNOTIC PARTS TECHNIQUE

Purpose: Gain information, resolve issues, or reach a goal.

Notes: This is a complex technique but powerful, so be patient. It's based upon *parts therapy* (see *Hypnosis For Inner Conflict Resolution* by Roy Hunter) and on *Six Step Reframing* (see *Frogs Into Princes* by Richard Bandler and John Grinder).

1. Sit quietly and think about the issue to resolve (or the goal to achieve). Listen to your thoughts.

2. Ask your subconscious mind a question.
- "Subconscious mind, there's a part of you that really understands this issue (or goal) of _____. Would it be alright for that part to come forward?"

3. Listen for an answer (usually yes or no).

4. When you receive an answer, thank your subconscious mind.
- "Subconscious mind, thank you for that answer."
- If "yes," go to the next step. If "no," then thank your subconscious and revisit the technique later that day.

5. Ask three questions to the part.
- "Part, thanks for stepping forward. What is your name?" Listen.
- "What's one benefit you get from [unwanted behavior/thought]?" Listen.
- "I understand you get benefit X. What does getting X do for you?" Listen.

6. Repeat the benefit questions until you're satisfied.

7. Then make an interesting offer.
- "I have an idea. You can get all those benefits [list them for the subconscious mind], plus more, by doing things

differently, in a healthier way. Are you interested in learning how?"

8. Listen for an answer.
- If "yes," then move on to the next step.
- If "no," then say, "I'm a bit puzzled. If you keep all the benefits and get new ones, it seems you'd want to know my idea. Would you like to at least hear the idea?" If still "no," then explain differently until it understands. With practice, you get better at this. After you get a "yes" go to step 9.

9. Ask the creative part to help create solutions.
- "That's great! Let's bring in the creative part to help us create possible solutions for you to choose from."
- "Creativity [or name you choose], your job is to come up with possible solutions. You needn't be concerned about good ideas versus bad ideas. Just give us ideas, and we'll decide which ones to keep. You're free to focus on ideas, just giving ideas."

10. Wait for a few answers from Creativity.
- "Thank you for those answers. Now, Part [named earlier], which of these answers do you like?"
- The part responds.
- "Thank you. Now if it's appropriate and healthy for all concerned, go ahead and let those solutions become a natural part of you. Let them absorb into you. When you feel you're finished, just say done."

11. Wait for it to say "done."
- "Thank you for all your help. If there's anything more that needs to be done, please let me know."
- If there is, discuss it. If not, you're done. Then gently allow yourself to come back to full consciousness. Slowly walk around, drink some water, and fully awaken yourself.

Example . . . Let's revisit Elizabeth and Party Liz.
See chapter three for a refresher. Let's observe how she uses the Hypnotic Parts Technique.

Steps 1–3: Elizabeth listens to her thoughts; her subconscious allows the part to step forward.
Elizabeth sits quietly and thinks about resolving the weight issue. She'd like to shed the excess pounds more easily and permanently, without struggle. She listens to her thoughts.

When she feels relaxed, she says, "Subconscious mind, there's a part of you that really understands my goal of losing weight easily, without struggle. Would it be alright for that part to come forward?" She listens and senses a "yes."

Step 4: She thanks her subconscious for the answer.
Elizabeth says, "Subconscious mind, thank you for that answer." Since it was a "yes," she can move on to step five.

Steps 5–6: She asks the part about benefits, repeating the questions until she feels satisfied.
Elizabeth: "Part, thanks for stepping forward. What's your name?" She listens for an answer.

Part: "I'm Party Liz."

Elizabeth: "Party Liz, it's nice to meet you. What's one benefit you get from me being kind of heavy?"

Party Liz: "I don't care about weight. I care about fun, eating tasty food, watching television, and relaxing, doing nothing."

Elizabeth: "Thank you for that answer. I understand that you have fun from all of that. What does having fun do for you?"

Party Liz: "What do you mean? Fun is fun."

Elizabeth: "What else does fun get for you or do for you? For example, if you have fun, maybe you get something else."

Party Liz: "I guess fun makes me feel good."

Elizabeth: "Yes! That's what I'm talking about. Fun makes you feel good! What does feeling good do for you or get for you?"

Party Liz: "Feeling good is just good."

Elizabeth: "Yes, I get that feeling good is good, and maybe something more. If so, what does feeling good get for you?"

Party Liz: "I feel good, comfortable. Is that what you mean?"

Elizabeth: "Yes! When you feel comfortable, what does that get for you or do for you?"

Party Liz: "I feel good. Oh, did we just go in a circle?"

Elizabeth: "That's okay! A circle's fine. So you feel comfortable and good. What does that get for you?"

Party Liz: "I guess I feel safe. Does that seem strange?"

Elizabeth: "No, not at all. Everyone likes to feel safe. What does feeling safe do for you or get for you?"

Party Liz: "I think that's all. I feel good, comfortable, and safe. It's all wrapped up together."

Steps 7–8: She makes an interesting offer.
Elizabeth: "Thank you for those answers. I have an idea. You can get all those benefits, such as fun, feeling good, feeling comfortable, and feeling safe. Plus you can get more benefits. And you can get all of this by doing things differently, in a healthier way. Are you interested in learning how?"

Party Liz: "Not really. I like things the way they are."

Elizabeth: "Change can be less comfortable than keeping things the same. Yet aren't you a little curious about how to keep all your benefits and get new benefits, too?"

Party Liz: "No. I'm happy with what I have."

Elizabeth: "I understand. Why change a good thing, right? Instead, how about if I say don't change anything right now. Instead, how about spending a bit of time learning something new? It may not affect anything today, but perhaps one day, way in the future, you might get something useful from what you learn today. I mean, haven't you ever learned something that came in handy much later? Has that ever happened?"

Party Liz: "Of course. Not everything's useful right now."

Elizabeth: "Yes, and some information may never be useful, right?"

Party Liz: "Yes."

Elizabeth: "Since we both agree on all of that, I have some information to share with you, information that may not be useful today and may not be useful in the future. But I can't really say either way, because only you can figure that out. It might be useful for you later, or maybe not. What do you think; do you have time to hear this information?"

Party Liz: "You're very persistent, aren't you?"

Elizabeth: "Yes I am! If I feel I can help you and me, I'm persistent. But only hear me out if you want to. If you don't, then just say so, because I don't want to pressure you."

Party Liz: "Okay, I guess I can at least hear you out."

Step 9: Creativity helps out.

Elizabeth: "Great! Before you hear the information, let's talk to the creative part to gain possible solutions to consider. Creative part, what may I call you?"

The new part: "Call me Creativity."

Elizabeth: "Creativity, welcome! Your job is to come up with possible solutions to the goal of getting to a healthy weight while still preserving fun, feeling good, comfortable, and safe. You needn't be concerned about good ideas versus bad ideas. Just give us ideas, and we'll decide which ones to consider. You're free to focus on ideas, just ideas. Make sense?"

Creativity: "Yes, it makes sense."

Elizabeth: "Then start coming up with ideas, now, and then let us know when you're ready to share."

Creativity: "Okay." Creativity thinks for a while.

Step 10: Creativity gives the answers.

Creativity: "I've got some answers. Do something fun, like taking a dance class with your husband. That'll improve your health and be fun and exciting."

Creativity: "Experiment with new and exotic recipes, maybe learn about Thai or Korean food, something different and tasty. That keeps calories down and is fun and feels good; I'm not sure about the comfortable and safe part, but this is part of an answer."

Creativity: "Look at this issue differently. In the short run, eating a lot and sitting on the couch might be fun, but later could lead to disease and pain. And that's not comfortable or safe! But you can prevent all that and feel more secure knowing that you're feeling good now and will feel good in the future."

Elizabeth: "Wow, Creativity, you gave great answers! Thank you! Party Liz, do any of these ideas interest you? Remember I'm not pressuring you into changing. I'm asking if any idea interests you."

Party Liz: "They all sound interesting to me. I'm not making promises to change anything, but they're all interesting, especially the part about what happens in the long run. I hadn't really cared about the future, but Creativity makes a good point. Yeah Elizabeth, I know you've told me about the future, but it didn't register until I heard Creativity say it."

Elizabeth: "I'm glad these ideas interest you. And it's fine that you're not making any promises to change anything. I understand that it may take time to let the thoughts settle. We can talk some more another day. I just want to say thanks for considering the ideas."

Elizabeth: "Now if it's appropriate and healthy for all parts concerned, go ahead and let these answers be considered over the next few days. No need to change anything now, just let these ideas be considered. When you feel this process has started, just say 'started' when that happens."

Step 11: Conclusion
Party Liz: "Started."

Elizabeth: "Thank you for all your help. If there's anything more that needs to be said, please let me know."

Party Liz: "I'm all set, nothing more to say."

Elizabeth thinks about her conversation.
Elizabeth eases back into full consciousness and writes down the highlights of her self-hypnosis. She notes her progress in speaking to her subconscious mind. She feels that soon, Party Liz will become a valuable partner in helping her reach a healthier weight and enjoying the process.

Elizabeth understands that all parts need to be kept.
Party Liz isn't separate or outside of herself. Party Liz is a part of Elizabeth as her arm or leg or her sense of humor. She understands all parts of herself are valuable and worthy.

Parts are like children, and she needs to nurture the parts and help resolve the conflicts between parts of herself. It's not about getting rid of a part; heck, that would be like getting rid of your children! That's not a good option!

It's about educating the part, helping it to gently change behavior and beliefs, so that she allows for internal harmony.

All parts are valuable and worth keeping, even if they seem to do things that appear negative. All parts can be educated by Elizabeth so they're more productive members of herself.

Helpful tips
This technique is a template, a guide. Here are some tips.
1. Be respectful, as if you're talking to a friend or child. Some parts are mature, but many are young.
2. Go with the flow. Be patient with yourself as you practice.
3. Soon you'll figure out what's true and what's false.

The subconscious can lie, mislead, or be ignorant of the truth. Yet it can give very useful information. With practice you're able to detect whether it's giving you truth, lies, or something in between.

But hey, the conscious mind can also lie, mislead, or say something in between. The conscious and subconscious can both be ignorant of the truth. Neither is 100% wise or honest. Neither is superior. Both play the roles of student and teacher.

When the two stop fighting and unite, you reach your goal faster.

TRANSFORM YOUR INNER CRITIC

Purpose: To transform your inner critic into a friend, helping cheer you on instead of holding you back.

Notes: Some people don't realize how harmful their internal language can be to their health and happiness. Once they realize what's happening, they're amazed at how much better life becomes once they've tamed their inner critic. This technique is an application of the Hypnotic Parts Technique.

1. Imagine your inner critic (internal voice) that seems to hold you back.
- It may say, "You're not good enough," or "You idiot, you shouldn't have done that!"
- Or it may say, "I'm not good enough," or "I'm an idiot, I shouldn't have done that."

2. Get a sense of where the internal voice is located.
- Is it in the body? If so, where?
- Is it outside the body? If so, where?
- Is it in a mental space, i.e., not in physical space?

3. Ask the voice for its name and positive intention.
- After it says its name and positive intention, say thank you, and say that you'd like to play a game.

4. Start the game by modifying the voice.
- Perhaps make it a silly cartoon voice.
- Or perhaps the voice of a famous actor.
- You decrease the emotional charge when you change the voice, so you may feel it's more neutral or humorous. For example, in real life if someone breathed in helium and had a high-pitched voice and yelled at you, you'd laugh instead of being upset.

5. Modify the voice even further.
- Experiment with the tone; make it a sexy voice, whiny voice, an accent, etc. Be creative!
- Experiment with speeding it up or slowing it down.
- Experiment with making it louder or softer.
- Experiment until you take the emotional charge out of the voice, so you feel it's neutral or humorous.

6. Move the voice to a silly place.
- Perhaps imagine the voice moving down to your big toe or some other silly place.

7. After you're done, offer the voice a new job.
- Say, "You've worked hard for years in your current job. You deserve a promotion! You can still get what you want; it's just that you'll get it more easily as my personal cheerleader. How does that sound?"
- Cheerleader is just an example. You and the voice may choose a different job for it. Listen for a response.
- If the voice agrees, say a few words about how you'd like it to be in its new role and thank it for accepting the new role. You might say, "Instead of criticizing me because you want me to perform better, help me prepare ahead of time so I do perform well."
- If the inner critic disagrees about getting promoted, use the Hypnotic Parts Technique to get to the bottom of things.

Example of Carla in remission from cancer.
But her inner critic still isn't satisfied with the great progress. Ironically, the critic doesn't realize that this criticism hinders Carla's progress. But the critic is about to get educated.

Step 1: Carla imagines her inner critic (internal voice) talking about her healthier lifestyle.
Voice: "You're eating healthy food, exercising, and using hypnosis to improve your health. But you're not doing enough. You need to double the amount of exercise within one week."

Step 2: She finds where the internal voice is located.
She senses it near her left shoulder and hears it in her left ear.

Step 3: She asks for its name and positive intention.
Carla: "I hear what you said about doubling my exercise within one week. What may I call you?"

Voice: "Just call me Speedy."

Carla: "Okay Speedy. What's your positive intention for me to increase my exercise?"

Speedy: "I'm in a hurry."

Carla: "Okay, what's useful about being in a hurry?"

Speedy: "I don't know if it's useful, but I'm just used to doing things quickly. It feels good. And I don't like slow people."

Carla: "Thank you for sharing that. I'd like to play a little game of pretend. You don't have to do too much, okay?"

Speedy: "Okay."

Step 4: Carla modifies Speedy's voice.
She changes it from deep, unfriendly, and masculine (with hints of a female voice) to Mickey Mouse's friendly voice.

Step 5: She modifies the voice even further.
She makes it a flirtatious Mickey Mouse voice; then adding a British accent; then an American Southern accent; finally deciding upon a flirtatious French accent since France is a favorite place for her. Now the voice is slow, soft, and playful.

Carla feels relaxed with this new voice. The emotional charge is almost all gone now that Speedy's talking in this new way.

Step 6: She moves the voice to a silly place.
Carla mentally moves the voice from her left shoulder area to her right thumb. Now the emotional charge is gone, and as she stares at her thumb, she begins laughing.

Step 7: She offers Speedy a new job.
Carla: "Speedy, you've worked hard over the years as the internal critic. You deserve a promotion! You can still get what you want, which is to feel good. It's just that you'll get to feel good by doing a different job. How does that sound?"

Speedy: "You mean I could be your health consultant, telling you what's potentially good and bad about a health idea? I'd like to help you figure things out."

Carla: "Yes, you could be my health consultant!"

Speedy: "I like that! I can read books and do research!"

Carla: "Great! So instead of pushing me to double my exercise so fast, you can help me research and evaluate my health options. What are the pros and cons of doing X, Y, or Z? You can help me evaluate options. How's that sound to you?"

Speedy: "That sounds really good! I like it!"

Carla: "Great! Thank you for all your past hard work, and I look forward to working with you in your new role."

Note about the inner critic's location

Remember that Carla's inner critic was located in her left shoulder area, and she hears it with her left ear. Sometimes location is unimportant, but in her case it might be important.

When Carla was growing up, her mother often criticized her. During meals, her mother sat to Carla's left, and would often say things such as, "You're such a slow eater. Why can't you hurry up? . . . You're too fat; you'd better exercise more young lady . . . You'd better marry a rich man, because you're not smart enough to make it on your own."

It's possible that Carla's subconscious mind absorbed some of her mother's viewpoints and began criticizing Carla just as her mother would. I'm not saying that all of this is true; it's just possible that she was greatly influenced by her mother. Or it could just be coincidence that her inner critic is located near her left shoulder area.

Helpful tip

Some readers might think that this technique can't possibly transform an inner critic into a friend. It might even seem silly. Well, it is, but that's okay! Give yourself permission to have fun with this technique. Let yourself experiment and have fun as you learn hypnosis.

I got frustrated on the first day of hypnosis school.

Our instructor hypnotized the class, but I didn't go deep into hypnosis. Then he had people share their experiences. One person talked about swimming with dolphins. Some talked about being so relaxed, and some even had profound spiritual experiences. I thought, "Darn it! How come I didn't go deep?"

The next day I still didn't go deep, so I had a chat with myself. "I'm in hypnosis school, and I'm not going deep. Is something wrong with me? Maybe I'm taking this too seriously. Maybe I need to stop trying so hard to enter hypnosis. Here's what I'll do. I'll take it easy on myself and see what happens."

As I stopped criticizing, I went out like a light.

The next group hypnosis I went so deep, so fast, that I only recall the instructor leading us back to awakening. Normally people remember what happened in hypnosis, but on that day, I forgot what happened. I went deep, and I felt great!

I realized that trying hard isn't the key to success.

I had to allow myself to succeed. Instead of working hard at these techniques, perhaps allow yourself to ease into learning hypnosis without judgment. Perhaps be kinder to yourself.

PART 3
HYPNOSIS SCRIPTS 101

Earlier you saw a few techniques. Now in part three we get to the heart of this book: hypnosis scripts. And in part four, you will have the opportunity to write your own script.

Here are the major topics in part three.
- Ch 8: Hypnosis Script Basics
- Ch 9: Overview: How to Write a Script
- Ch 10: Jane's Step-by-Step Script Generator

By the way, I mentioned in part one to skim this book instead of reading it in great detail, at least on your first time reading this book. Then when you read the book a second time, it'll be easier to understand.

Well, skimming is especially important with parts three and four. Skim these chapters on hypnosis scripts the first time through. For now, hold off on actually using hypnosis scripts.

Then on the second time through this book, you'll be able to absorb these concepts and then begin using these techniques. Bottom line: please skim now, and hold off on writing a script until the second time reading this book.

"I have an almost complete disregard of precedent, and a faith in the possibility of something better. It irritates me to be told how things have always been done. I defy the tyranny of precedent. I go for anything new that might improve the past."

Clara Barton
Founder of the American Red Cross

CH 8: HYPNOSIS SCRIPT BASICS

In this chapter, we'll answer these questions.
- "What is a hypnosis script?"
- "What do I gain from creating my own hypnosis script?"
- "Is there any downside to creating my own hypnosis script?"
- "What does a hypnosis script look like?"
- "What about 'you' versus 'I' language?"

"WHAT IS A HYPNOSIS SCRIPT?"

It's a set of suggestions written on paper. Here are the steps.

- Write the script.
- Read the script out loud to record it.
- Listen to the recording as often as needed.

Recording lengths vary, say from 10-30 minutes. Each time you listen, you're hypnotizing yourself and strengthening the suggestions in your subconscious. Then you let go of blocks faster and reach your goal faster.

"WHAT DO I GAIN FROM CREATING MY OWN HYPNOSIS SCRIPT?"

It helps you reach your goal more quickly and more easily.

Sure, commercial hypnosis script recordings can be bought, and some work well. But they're not customized to you.

By learning how to create your own script, you customize to your situation, and that increases its power. It requires work to become skilled at it, but in my opinion, it's worth it.

Besides health-related goals, you can use scripts to improve your career, make more money, strengthen relationships, improve sports performance, etc. It's a flexible tool, plus it's cheaper than hiring a hypnotherapist.

"IS THERE ANY DOWNSIDE TO CREATING MY OWN HYPNOSIS SCRIPT?"

In rare cases, yes.

If someone writes a bad script, usually the worst that happens is that the script simply doesn't work, meaning that the person isn't any worse off than before.

For health issues, it's wise to understand the health issue in more detail so you can write a comprehensive script, thus avoiding any potential pitfalls.

Let's say that John just had knee surgery and wants to heal faster. He writes a hypnosis script to accelerate the healing of his leg. He writes about his leg being flexible and able to easily walk up and down stairs. Sounds good, right?

Well, flexibility is only one part of the equation; strengthening muscles also makes walking stairs possible. His script missed at least one important element, and possibly more.

That's why it's crucial to view the issue in a comprehensive way. That may even include showing the script to a health professional.

John talks to his physical therapist and says, "I want to heal faster. My script focuses on flexibility. Is there more that I should focus upon? Am I missing some element?" Then his physical therapist explains about strengthening and whatever else is important in John's case.

Bottom line: do your homework by understanding the health issue, so you can create a more comprehensive script. And think about showing it to your health professional to ensure that you covered all the important points. Even if they aren't familiar with hypnosis, you can still get their advice on what's important to healing quickly.

"WHAT DOES A HYPNOSIS SCRIPT LOOK LIKE?"

On the next few pages is a sample script titled *Gain My Freedom*. It's about smoking cessation. Rather than analyzing it deeply, I suggest briefly skimming it. If the wording or grammar seems unusual, I did it on purpose to deepen hypnosis more quickly.

The words in brackets in the script are descriptions to make it easier to follow. You would not read those words out loud.

GAIN MY FREEDOM

(Subject is smoking cessation; unusual wording deepens hypnosis.)

[Stage 1: Relaxation]

Go ahead and ease into a comfortable position with your eyes open. In a few moments, you'll be closing your eyes and taking a nice little break just for yourself. So you may want to turn off the phone and close the door, so you can have a relaxed and restful time.

If for some reason you need to get up during this program, you will easily come out of hypnosis and take care of whatever needs to be done. And when you return to the program from where you left off a few moments ago, you'll find that you may easily get back into that very relaxed state you were already in, or even find yourself instantly being more relaxed than before.

Remember, this is your time, when you do something good just for yourself. Go ahead and close your eyes, relax, and feel good. You deserve this time for yourself. As you relax deeply, you'll receive positive suggestions to help you . . . So go ahead and relax deeply . . .

Right now, during this program, all you need to do is simply breathe, relax, and listen to this program. Your to-do list can wait. Other people can wait. Other thoughts can wait. This is your time to go deep . . . now is your time to spend just with yourself.

As I count from 10 to 1, let yourself become more relaxed, naturally, easily, and at your own pace.
10, . . . deeper relaxed . . . 9, . . . deeper relaxed . . .
8, . . . deeper relaxed . . . 7, . . . deeper relaxed . . .
6, . . . deeper relaxed . . . 5, . . . deeper relaxed . . .
4, . . . deeper relaxed . . . 3, . . . deeper relaxed . . .
2, . . . deeper relaxed . . . 1, . . . deeper relaxed . . .

[Stage 2: Suggestions]

[Goal]
I gain my freedom from nicotine, because I care about my grandchildren, my family, and myself. In the past, it was tough to quit smoking, because I only used will power. But now I realize that will power isn't the key, because will power is a tool of the conscious mind. But smoking is a type of habit, and it's controlled by the subconscious mind.

To change a habit, I need to speak to the one in charge of it, and that's you subconscious mind! So subconscious mind, I ask you for help. Help me let go of that old behavior of smoking, and replace it with something better, which is freedom! United, we succeed!

[Benefit A]
By gaining my freedom, I spend more time with my grandchildren, not having to worry about harming them with second-hand smoke or the smoke from my clothes. This is important to me, because they grow up so fast! I want to see them as much as I can while they're young!

And I definitely want to see my grandchildren grow up to be wonderful adults. Subconscious mind, gaining my freedom helps me stay healthy. By staying healthy, my family won't have to worry about my health. Instead, they can focus on their own lives and be happier. And of course I'll be happier staying healthy, too!

[Benefit B]
Gaining my freedom makes my clothes and body smell fresh and clean. I miss feeling clean, and I want that feeling back! It's important to me! Smelling and feeling clean gives me more confidence. I feel more comfortable in my own skin. It just feels good!

In the long term, feeling good is just good. I can't say more than that. Feeling good just feels good! And for my family and friends, when I smell clean, they're more comfortable and happier, too! And that makes me happy. I mean, I'm gaining my freedom because I care about me, and I'm doing this because I care about my family.

[Benefit C]
And last but not least, I want to let go of coughing and breathe freely. Breathing freely and easily just makes me feel good! Most people take it for granted, but I don't. I cherish being able to breathe freely and easily.

Breathing freely and easily just makes my life better in so many ways. I can walk to the store without a problem. And I can walk up a flight of stairs and feel fine. I'll be able to get through the day with my throat feeling good and be able to sleep through the night easily.

In the long term, good health makes my life happier. And I definitely want my life to be happier. By improving my health right now, I'll be happier today and tomorrow. By taking care of myself, I'll be happier. And when I'm happier, my family and friends will be happier, because my life affects their lives. And I care about their happiness.

[Summary]
So subconscious mind, to gain my freedom, I need your help. Gaining my freedom means I get to spend more time with my grandchildren, and that's important for them and for me. They grow up so fast!

Gaining my freedom makes my clothes and body smell fresh and clean. And I want that feeling back! It's important to me! Gaining my freedom means I can breathe freely and easily, and that just makes me feel good! I cherish breathing freely and easily.

Let's keep taking action until I gain my freedom, because I care about my grandchildren, my family and friends, and last but not least, I care about my happiness! And because I care so much about me, I want to live a long and happy life.

And if that means letting go of smoking and gaining my freedom, then I'll do that! Thank you for helping me gain my freedom!

[Stage 3: Awakening]
I will count from 5 to 1. With each number counted, let everything you've learned in this program go deeper and deeper into your subconscious, allowing what you have learned to become a part of who you are. 5, 4, 3, 2, 1.

In a few moments, this program will be ending, and you'll be ready to gently come back to a fully conscious state of mind. I'll soon count from 1 to 10. With each number counted, let yourself become more alert, awake, and refreshed.

1, feel what's beneath your body, perhaps a bed, chair, or floor.
2, let yourself become more alert.
3, let yourself feel more awake.
4, feeling more refreshed.
5, feel the air in the room.
6, let your body become restless, wanting to get up soon.
7, feel the energy rushing gently back into your body.
8, feel yourself really wanting to become fully conscious.
9, feel even more alert, awake, and refreshed.
And 10, when you're ready, you may open your eyes, stand up, and stretch, feeling very alert, awake, and refreshed, as if you've gotten up from a nice nap.

Simply feeling good . . . simply feeling good . . . simply feeling good.

"WHAT ABOUT 'YOU' VERSUS 'I' LANGUAGE?"

You may've noticed that the relaxation and awakening stages used the word "you." And the middle stage (suggestions stage) used the word "I."

That's just one of three approaches. Some people only use "I" or only use "you" in their script. Of these three approaches, which is best? Is it best to mix the pronouns or stay only with one of them?

It's what works for you. When I write for myself, and I'm the only one who'll hear it, I use "you" in all three stages. But that's my preference. When it comes to hypnosis, so much depends upon the individual. Experiment and find out what works best for you.

CHAPTER REVIEW

"What is a hypnosis script?"
It's a set of suggestions written down on paper. Usually you'd read the script and record it for future listening.

"What do I gain from creating my own hypnosis script?"
You can reach your goal more quickly and more easily. It's customized to your needs.

"Is there any downside to creating my own hypnosis script?"
If someone writes a bad script, rarely are there negative effects. Usually the worst that'll happen is the script simply doesn't work.

"What does a hypnosis script look like?"
We briefly skimmed a sample script, *Gain My Freedom*.

"What about 'you' versus 'I' language?"
There are three approaches: 'you' or 'I' or a combination. Use what works for you.

- -

Next we'll look at the overview of how to write a script.

"I am an optimist. It does not seem too much use being anything else."

Winston Churchill
British Prime Minster

CH 9: OVERVIEW:
HOW TO WRITE A SCRIPT

In this chapter, we'll look at these topics.
- "What are the four big steps to writing a script?"
- "State the goal in the positive? What's that?"
- "What's a negative suggestion?"
- "How do you state a goal in the positive?"
- "Can you give an example of a positive goal for a hypnosis script?"
- "Can you say more about the three stages?"

"WHAT ARE THE FOUR BIG STEPS TO WRITING A SCRIPT?"

1. State the goal in the positive.
2. Create the relaxation stage.
3. Create the suggestions stage.
4. Create the awakening stage.

"STATE THE GOAL IN THE POSITIVE? WHAT'S THAT?"

When you write a script, you can use negative suggestions or positive suggestions. In my opinion, having more positive suggestions works better. Let's first define negative suggestion.

"WHAT'S A NEGATIVE SUGGESTION?"

A negative suggestion tells you what not to do. Let's do an experiment. Inhale deeply . . . and exhale gently. Then follow the next suggestion: "Don't think of a pink elephant."

Most will think of a pink elephant. Are they being difficult? No, they're trying to follow my suggestion, trying not to think about the pink elephant. But that's tough to do, because the brain has to think about the elephant first in order to not think about the elephant. The more effort, the worse the result.

Here's another: George just got fired from his job. His friend Jerry visits to cheer him up and says, "George, don't think about getting fired. It's over, so why think about it?" All night Jerry keeps telling George not to think about the firing. Each time Jerry brings up the suggestion helps keep George stuck.

In other words, negative suggestions have a downside. The subconscious finds it tougher to process *what not to do*. It's easier to process *what to do*. Here are examples of negative language.
- Don't
- Won't
- Can't
- Shouldn't
- Stop

By telling the subconscious what to avoid, or stop doing, the subconscious may get confused. The subconscious finds it easier to process positive suggestions, not negatives ones.

Why distinguish between negative and positive suggestions? You want your subconscious to help you. So give it more of the easy-to-follow suggestions (i.e., positive suggestions). I'm not saying to avoid all negative suggestions. Done right, negative language patterns can be useful. But when you're starting out with hypnosis, stick with positive suggestions.

"HOW DO YOU STATE A GOAL IN THE POSITIVE?"

State what you *do want* rather than what you *don't want*. Using the pink elephant as an example, if you don't want your friend Seth to think of a pink elephant, say it differently.

Instead of saying, "Seth, don't think of a pink elephant," say, "Seth, think of a purple cow." Now your friend Seth will focus on the purple cow. By telling him what to focus upon, he's more likely to do it. Your positive suggestion makes it clear what you want him to do.

Mrs. Butterworth's flower bed gets trampled!

Let's say you're babysitting a friend's five-year-old child. You both walk by Mrs. Butterworth's house, your sweet neighbor. The child walks into the garden, destroying flowers.

A negative suggestion doesn't work so well.

Many would say, "Stop walking on the flowers!" But have you noticed that when you tell a child to stop doing something, she'll stop only to start up again? The subconscious has a tough time with negative suggestions.

But a positive suggestion works better!

You say, "Mrs. Butterworth will feel sad if her flowers get stepped on. It's better to let the flowers grow. Let's walk on the sidewalk, because that's the better place to walk."

Instead of telling the child *what not to do,* you're letting her focus on *what to do.* When we focus on *what to do,* it's easier to do it. Children learn faster and understand clearly when we give positive suggestions. The subconscious is like a child, so we can use this principle in self-hypnosis for ourselves!

"CAN YOU GIVE AN EXAMPLE OF A POSITIVE GOAL FOR A HYPNOSIS SCRIPT?"

Jane says, "I want to quit smoking."

Jane's goal above is stated in the negative.

She says what she doesn't want, meaning she doesn't want to smoke. That's a tougher goal for the subconscious to strive for *not doing*. Let's convert her goal into a positive goal.

Let's ask Jane for her benefits from quitting smoking.

- She wants to spend time with her grandkids without harming them through smoking.
- She wants to get rid of the smell of smoke from her clothes and body; or to say it positively, she wants to smell fresh and clean.
- Instead of coughing and being a slave to nicotine, she wants to breathe freely and be in control of her body.
- Instead of feeling ashamed of her addiction, she wants to feel proud of herself for gaining her freedom.

Bottom line: she wants to gain her freedom from nicotine, because she'll get all those benefits listed; they satisfy her emotionally. The surface goal is about smoking, but her deeper goal is to gain those benefits listed.

Jane's goal is now restated in the positive.

"I gain my freedom, because I care about my grandchildren and myself."

Notice she says *gain my freedom*. It's a more emotionally attractive goal to her than quitting smoking. Her new goal directs her subconscious mind to what she wants instead of what she doesn't want. You can see her script in the previous chapter with the script titled *Gain My Freedom*.

"CAN YOU SAY MORE ABOUT THE THREE STAGES?"

Before talking about the three stages, let's review. We've discussed the difference between a negative suggestion and a positive suggestion. The subconscious mind has an easier time processing positive suggestions than negative ones.

We saw Jane convert a negative goal into a positive goal by getting to the heart of what she truly wants. By giving voice to her true desires, she crafted a goal she can truly feel good about, and that helps her achieve it. Now let's go to the three stages.

In the first question of this chapter, I mentioned the four big steps to writing a script, and three stages were part of those four steps. Here's a bit more detail about the three stages.

After you decide upon your goal, you would structure your script. A script contains three distinct stages.
1. Relaxation stage (you gently ease yourself into hypnosis)
2. Suggestions stage (you give yourself reasons why your goal is worth achieving; get your subconscious excited about success)
3. Awakening stage (you gently ease yourself out of hypnosis and back to a fully conscious state)

For your first script, we'll use a generic relaxation stage and a generic awakening stage. That means you'll only need to write one of the three stages.

CHAPTER REVIEW

"What are the four big steps to writing a script?"
1. State the goal in the positive.
2. Create the relaxation stage.
3. Create the suggestions stage.
4. Create the awakening stage.

"State the goal in the positive? What's that?"
There are negative and positive suggestions. First let's define negative suggestion.

"What's a negative suggestion?"
A negative suggestion tells you what not to do. For example, "Don't think of a pink elephant." The subconscious has a tougher time processing *what not to do.*

"How do you state a goal in the positive?"
State what you want instead of what you don't want. Instead of saying, "Seth, don't think of a pink elephant," say, "Seth, think of a purple cow."

"Can you give an example of a positive goal for a hypnosis script?"
Jane's goal went from a negative goal, "I want to quit smoking," to "I gain my freedom, because I care about my grandchildren and myself."

"Can you say more about the three stages?"
After you decide upon your goal, you would structure your script. A script contains three distinct stages.
1. Relaxation stage
2. Suggestions stage
3. Awakening stage

- -

Next Jane uses the step-by-step script generator.

"We will either find a way, or make one."

Hannibal
Ancient military general of Carthage

CH 10: JANE'S STEP-BY-STEP SCRIPT GENERATOR

Let's revisit Jane and her journey to gain her freedom from cigarettes. You'll see Jane fill out the step-by-step script generator, which is simply a series of questions divided into five major steps. After she fills it out, she'll have a rough draft for her hypnosis script.

We'll cover these topics.
- Step 1: Jane states her goal.
- Steps 2–4: Jane lists her benefits of reaching her goal.
- Step 5: Jane summarizes the benefits.
- Notes about Jane's script.

After you finish this chapter, you'll have the opportunity to fill out your own script generator!

Step 1: State your goal in the positive.

A. State the goal.

I gain my freedom from nicotine, because I care about my grandchildren and myself.

B. If appropriate, mention why it was difficult to achieve your goal in the past, and why things are different now (i.e., you're using hypnosis, so that will make things easier; and/or something else has changed).

In the past, it was tough to quit smoking, because I tried using will power. But now things are different, because I understand will power isn't the answer. Now I understand that my subconscious mind holds the key to my freedom.

I understand that smoking is a habit, and that my subconscious mind stores habits. That's why I now speak directly to my subconscious mind by using this hypnosis script.

And I ask my subconscious mind to help me to gain my freedom.

Step 2: Describe major benefit A.

A. State a compelling benefit that drives you to reach your goal.

By gaining my freedom, I spend more time with my grandchildren, not having to worry about harming them with second-hand smoke or the smoke from my clothes.

B. Why is this benefit so compelling to you in the short term?

This is important to me, because they grow up so fast! I want to see them as much as I can while they're young!

C. Why is this benefit so compelling to you in the long term?

In the long term, I want to see my grandchildren grow up to be wonderful adults. And I can only do this by staying healthy. And by gaining my freedom, I'll help myself stay healthy.

D. Why is this benefit also good for others you care about?

By staying healthy, my family won't have to worry about me. They can focus on their own lives and be happier.

And of course I'll be happier staying healthy, too!

Step 3: Describe major benefit B.

A. State a compelling benefit that drives you to reach your goal.

Gaining my freedom makes my clothes and body smell fresh and clean. I miss feeling clean, and I want that feeling back! It's important to me!

B. Why is this benefit so compelling to you in the short term?

Smelling and feeling clean gives me more confidence. I feel more comfortable in my own skin. It just feels good!

C. Why is this benefit so compelling to you in the long term?

In the long term, feeling good is just good. I can't say more than that. Feeling good just feels good!

D. Why is this benefit also good for others you care about?

For my family and friends, when I smell clean, they're more comfortable and happier, too! And that makes me happy. I mean, I'm gaining my freedom because I care about me, and I'm doing this because I care about my family.

Step 4: Describe major benefit C.

A. State a compelling benefit that drives you to reach your goal.

I want to let go of coughing and breathe freely.

Breathing freely and easily just makes me feel good! Most people take it for granted, but I don't. I cherish being able to breathe freely and easily.

B. Why is this benefit so compelling to you in the short term?

Breathing freely and easily just makes my life better in so many ways. I can walk to the store without a problem. I can walk up a flight of stairs and feel fine. It matters to me and will make my life better.

C. Why is this benefit so compelling to you in the long term?

In the long term, good health makes my life happier. And I definitely want my life to be happier. By improving my health right now, I'll be happier today and tomorrow.

D. Why is this benefit also good for others you care about?

By taking care of myself, I'll be happier. And when I'm happier, my family and friends will be happier, because my life affects their lives. And I care about their happiness.

> **Step 5: Briefly summarize why you're so motivated to succeed.**

A. Why is benefit A so great for you and others?

To wrap up, gaining my freedom means I get to spend more time with my grandchildren, and that's important for them and for me. They grow up so fast!

B. Why is benefit B so great for you and others?

Gaining my freedom makes my clothes and body smell fresh and clean. And I want that feeling back! It's important to me!

C. Why is benefit C so great for you and others?

Gaining my freedom means I can breathe freely and easily, and that just makes me feel good! I cherish breathing freely and easily.

D. Briefly explain why you'll keep going until you've succeeded.

I'll keep taking action until I gain my freedom, because I care about my grandchildren, my family and friends, and last but not least, I care about my own happiness!

And because I care so much about me, I want to live a long and happy life. And if that means letting go of smoking and gaining my freedom, then that's what I'll do!

NOTES ABOUT JANE'S SCRIPT

We've seen how Jane filled out the script generator. Her answers were the basis for her script, *Gain My Freedom,* back in chapter eight.

If you compare the script generator answers to her script, you'll see it's almost identical, except I labeled each script section in brackets so you can easily follow along. I labeled the first part *goal,* then I put the label of *benefit,* and then I put the label of *summary.*

Those labels (in bolded brackets) serve as a visual aid to know where you're at as you read a script. When you record a script, obviously you wouldn't read the bracketed labels out loud.

Of the three stages, relaxation, suggestions, and awakening, Jane only wrote the suggestions stage. It's the most important one, because it's customized to each person. The relaxation and awakening stages are generic, so feel free to use the ones provided in this book or modify to your preference.

CHAPTER REVIEW

Let's review where we're at. We've seen how Jane filled out the script generator.
- Step 1: Jane states her goal.
- Steps 2–4: Jane lists her benefits of reaching her goal.
- Step 5: Jane summarizes the benefits.
- Notes about Jane's script.

- -

In the next chapter, it's your turn to write your first draft!

PART 4
YOUR TURN TO WRITE A SCRIPT

You've just learned a few basics on writing a script. And you saw Jane fill out the step-by-step script generator. Now it's your turn to write your script.

Here are the topics in part four.
- Ch 11: Step-by-Step Script Generator
- Ch 12: Recording Your First Script

"Faith is taking the first step even when you don't see the whole staircase."

Martin Luther King, Jr.
Minister, American civil rights leader

CH 11: STEP-BY-STEP SCRIPT GENERATOR

While teaching script-writing to my students, I saw a pattern. The one who labored for hours to write a perfect first draft didn't learn as quickly as the one who spent minutes.

In script-writing, the hard worker has a disadvantage. That's why I recommend you spend as little time as possible on your first draft, meaning 30 minutes at the most.

This is the time to let your subconscious express itself, not a time for perfectionism, because perfectionism can hinder creativity and enjoyment.

Are you tempted to edit for spelling, grammar, and clarity? Skip all that. Doing a quick first draft is key.

For your first script, you'll be given a generic relaxation stage and a generic awakening stage. Since two of the three stages have been written, you'll save a lot of time. The suggestions stage is the most important stage, and that's our focus.

In this chapter, you'll write your script by doing the following:
- Use the generic relaxation stage given to you.
- State your goal in the positive.
- Describe major benefits of achieving your goal.
- Summarize the major benefits of achieving your goal.
- Use the generic awakening stage given to you.

Ready to write your first draft? Then let's go to the next page!

RELAXATION STAGE

Below, the relaxation stage is already here for you. Just take a quick look at it, and then go to the next page.

[Stage 1: Relaxation]

Go ahead and ease into a comfortable position with your eyes open. In a few moments, you'll be closing your eyes and taking a nice little break just for yourself. So you may want to turn off the phone and close the door, so you can have a relaxed and restful time.

If for some reason you need to get up during this program, you will easily come out of hypnosis and take care of whatever needs to be done. And when you return to the program from where you left off a few moments ago, you'll find that you may easily get back into that very relaxed state you were already in, or even find yourself instantly being more relaxed than before.

Remember, this is your time, when you do something good just for yourself. Go ahead and close your eyes, relax, and feel good. You deserve this time for yourself. As you relax deeply, you'll receive positive suggestions to help you . . . So go ahead and relax deeply . . .

Right now, during this program, all you need to do is simply breathe, relax, and listen to this program. Your to-do list can wait. Other people can wait. Other thoughts can wait. This is your time to go deep . . . now is your time to spend just with yourself.

As I count from 10 to 1, let yourself become more relaxed, naturally, easily, and at your own pace.
10, . . . deeper relaxed . . . 9, . . . deeper relaxed . . .
8, . . . deeper relaxed . . . 7, . . . deeper relaxed . . .
6, . . . deeper relaxed . . . 5, . . . deeper relaxed . . .
4, . . . deeper relaxed . . . 3, . . . deeper relaxed . . .
2, . . . deeper relaxed . . . 1, . . . deeper relaxed . . .

SUGGESTIONS STAGE

As discussed earlier, you'll only write the suggestions stage. Here's the outline to writing the suggestions stage.

1. State your goal in the positive.
2. Describe major benefit A.
3. Describe major benefit B.
4. Describe major benefit C.
5. Briefly summarize why you're so motivated to succeed.

Note about the blank lines on the script generator

The blank lines aren't a guide for how long to write your answers. You can write as much or as little as you'd like. I'd recommend getting out some blank paper so you have plenty of room to write your answers from the script generator.

If you're unsure of what to write, that's okay. Just write whatever comes to your mind. Act as if you didn't really care about the script. Doing it this way for your first draft helps to let your thoughts flow freely.

The script generator may look familiar, because you saw Jane fill it out in the previous chapter.

So get your timer set for 30 minutes and have some blank paper. Now start your timer and turn to the next page to start writing!

Step 1: State your goal in the positive.

A. State the goal.

_____

_____

B. If appropriate, mention why it was difficult to achieve your goal in the past, and why things are different now (i.e., you're using hypnosis, so that will make things easier; and/or something else has changed).

_____

_____

_____

_____

_____

_____

Step 2: Describe major benefit A.

A. State a compelling benefit that drives you to reach your goal.

_____

_____

B. Why is this benefit so compelling to you in the short term?

_____

_____

_____

C. Why is this benefit so compelling to you in the long term?

_____

_____

_____

D. Why is this benefit also good for others you care about?

_____

_____

_____

Step 3: Describe major benefit B.

A. State a compelling benefit that drives you to reach your goal.

_____

_____

B. Why is this benefit so compelling to you in the short term?

_____

_____

_____

C. Why is this benefit so compelling to you in the long term?

_____

_____

_____

D. Why is this benefit also good for others you care about?

_____

_____

_____

Step 4: Describe major benefit C.

A. State a compelling benefit that drives you to reach your goal.

_____

_____

B. Why is this benefit so compelling to you in the short term?

_____

_____

_____

C. Why is this benefit so compelling to you in the long term?

_____

_____

_____

D. Why is this benefit also good for others you care about?

_____

_____

_____

Step 5: Briefly summarize why you're so motivated to succeed.

A. Why is benefit A so great for you and others?

_____

_____

_____

B. Why is benefit B so great for you and others?

_____

_____

_____

C. Why is benefit C so great for you and others?

_____

_____

_____

D. Briefly explain why you'll keep going until you've succeeded.

_____

_____

_____

AWAKENING STAGE

Congratulations! You've just finished writing the foundation of your suggestions stage! You were given the relaxation stage. And below you've been given the awakening stage.

You now have all three stages written! In the next chapter, you'll do something with your script. After you briefly skim the awakening stage below, go to the next page.

[Stage 3: Awakening]

I will count from 5 to 1. With each number counted, let everything you've learned in this program go deeper and deeper into your subconscious, allowing what you have learned to become a part of who you are. 5, 4, 3, 2, 1.

In a few moments, this program will be ending, and you'll be ready to gently come back to a fully conscious state of mind. I'll soon count from 1 to 10. With each number counted, let yourself become more alert, awake, and refreshed.

1, feel what's beneath your body, perhaps a bed, chair, or floor.
2, let yourself become more alert.
3, let yourself feel more awake.
4, feeling more refreshed.
5, feel the air in the room.
6, let your body become restless, wanting to get up soon.
7, feel the energy rushing gently back into your body.
8, feel yourself really wanting to become fully conscious.
9, feel even more alert, awake, and refreshed.
And 10, when you're ready, you may open your eyes, stand up, and stretch, feeling very alert, awake, and refreshed, as if you've gotten up from a nice nap.

Simply feeling good . . . simply feeling good . . . simply feeling good.

CHAPTER REVIEW

Let's review where we're at.
- You have a generic relaxation stage.
- You've stated your goal in the positive.
- You've written its major compelling benefits.
- You've summarized those benefits.
- You have a generic awakening stage.

Though the suggestions stage you've written may not look like a script, you've just created the foundation of what will become your first script! Give yourself a pat on the back, because you've just done something few people ever do: you wrote your first hypnosis script. It may be a first draft, but it's still a script!

- -

Next let's record your first script!

CH 12: RECORDING YOUR FIRST SCRIPT

Let's answer a few questions in this chapter, and after this chapter you'll be able to record your first script.

- "Is it dangerous to listen while driving?"
- "When do I listen to my script? How often?"
- "Can I aim for multiple goals, or should I stick to one?"
- "How do I speak as I record my script?"
- "What equipment do I need to record my script?"
- "Since I began practicing self-hypnosis, I've noticed good things happening to me. Is this a coincidence?"
- "What if I'm not healing quickly? Am I missing a step?"

Now you may be wondering if it's better to revise your script before recording it. After all, it's only a rough draft right now.

Normally, that's good advice. But I've observed that my best students were the ones who recorded their first draft quickly. That's why I recommend recording your first script now, and then revising it later if needed.

"IS IT DANGEROUS TO LISTEN WHILE DRIVING?"
Yes, it's dangerous to listen to a script while driving or doing anything active. Listen in a quiet place, with your eyes closed.

"WHEN DO I LISTEN TO MY SCRIPT? HOW OFTEN?"
Listening in the morning sets a good tone for the day, but it's your decision. Whatever you do, I recommend a routine.
1. Listen at the same time each day.
2. Or link your script to an existing routine. For example, if you jog at 8:00 AM, link jogging to your script so that after you jog, you listen to your script. Linking makes it easier to create a habit.

Listen once a day until you don't need it. If you'd like to listen more often, that's fine, but once a day is good for most. It's tough to predict how many days/weeks to listen. My unofficial rule is to listen for two weeks before making any changes.

My friend couldn't leave his house without flossing.
When I told my friend that I was going to create a hypnosis CD to help people enjoy brushing and flossing, he volunteered to test it out. Afterwards he said, "I listened to your dental CD only once, and now I can't leave the house without flossing!"

Let me be clear that the CD was not forcing him to floss. He simply felt a strong desire to floss, especially before leaving home. But he still had the choice of whether to floss. It simply became easier to floss versus not to floss. It felt better!

Bottom line: he achieved his goal quickly. You may wonder why he only needed to listen to the CD once. I think he probably didn't have a big internal conflict about flossing. But if he had a big conflict, maybe he'd have needed to listen several times.

"CAN I AIM FOR MULTIPLE GOALS, OR SHOULD I STICK TO ONE?"

To keep things simple for now, I suggest focusing on one main goal in a script, and just use one script.

"HOW DO I SPEAK AS I RECORD MY SCRIPT?"

You may remember that each script has three stages.
1. Relaxation (ease yourself into hypnosis)
2. Suggestions (helps you reach your goal)
3. Awakening (helps you become fully conscious)

Here are duration guidelines and tips on how to speak.

Relaxation Stage
- Speak slowly, in a relaxed way.
- Speak with moderate volume and moderate emotion.
- Record for five to ten minutes.

Suggestions Stage
- Speak a bit faster.
- Speak a bit louder, with more enthusiasm.
- Remember that your subconscious is like a ten-year-old child. Convince it that your goal is worthy. Speak with logic, sincerity, and powerful emotion. Speak from your heart on why your goal is important and why the subconscious needs to help.
- Record for five to ten minutes.

Awakening Stage
- Speak a bit faster.
- Speak a bit louder with moderate to excited emotion.
- Record for one to three minutes.

"Awakening" isn't an accurate term, because you weren't asleep. But it's commonly used. After you "awaken," briefly walk and drink water to become fully conscious faster. The awakening stage helps prevents a foggy feeling after hypnosis.

"WHAT EQUIPMENT DO I NEED TO RECORD MY SCRIPT?"

There are three main ways to record your script.

Record with a computer.

You'll need a microphone and audio software. Most people can create a CD with the software included on their computer. Many computers have mp3 software to create mp3 recordings if you prefer an mp3 over a CD. If you don't find the right software on your computer, ask a technical friend for help. Or download free software from the Internet.

Record with a digital recorder.

This is the easiest way to record if you'd rather not use a computer. Plus the sound quality can be excellent.

Record with a cassette recorder.

This is my least favorite method, because the sound quality is mediocre. But you can boost sound quality with an external microphone.

"SINCE I BEGAN PRACTICING SELF-HYPNOSIS, I'VE NOTICED GOOD THINGS HAPPENING TO ME. IS THIS A COINCIDENCE?"

Many clients tell me about unexpected positive changes after practicing self-hypnosis. I believe that this is a ripple effect related to making one positive change. Somehow they attract, or create, these additional surprising positive changes. It has happened to me, too. Why does it happen? I'm not sure. I just tell clients to enjoy the unexpected benefits.

"WHAT IF I'M NOT HEALING QUICKLY? AM I MISSING A STEP?"

The answer's complex and could fill a book. Here are a few thoughts. Some heal faster, and it's not always predictable who's who. Some have complex issues that hinder healing. Or it might be that a person just needs a bit more time.

Here are a few factors that affect healing.
- Skill at using hypnosis (with practice, people improve)
- Type of hypnosis used
- Motivation level (the higher the better; does the person have a compelling reason to heal quickly?)
- Persistence (will the person do whatever it takes to heal, or is the person easily frustrated; if easily frustrated, it may be useful to strengthen their persistence through hypnosis)
- Complexity of the health condition
- Synergy of their healing plan (i.e., healthy diet, exercise, other healing modalities, and self-hypnosis)
- Support from friends and family (if a loved one is unsupportive about the health plan, in some cases that may hinder healing)

A few complex issues that may hinder healing
1. Anger and forgiveness
2. Fear
3. Self-worth
4. Identifying with a loved one

These complex issues can be tough to handle for someone new to self-hypnosis. If you suspect a complex issue, seek help from a hypnotherapist. In some cases, the hypnotherapist may refer you to a psychotherapist, or it may be good to work with both professionals.

As an example, forgiveness is a fairly common issue. I've helped many clients to forgive, and after they forgive, they release a lot of negative energy that's been pent up inside. After that, they tend to become happier and healthier.

This section on complex issues may be controversial to some. I'm not saying that this is the gospel when it comes to health issues. It's simply based upon what I've observed and learned from others. Remember that everyone's situation is unique.

1. Anger and forgiveness

If someone hangs onto anger toward someone, this may sometimes hinder the body from healing. Anger can be like acid, slowly eating away at a person. Forgiveness is about protecting yourself, to stop the acid from eating you. Don't forgive for their sake; forgive because you care about your own healing. Do it for you, not them.

A client grew up in an abusive home. As an adult, she suffered from major personal and health problems.

During hypnosis she chose to forgive her father for the many mistakes he'd made. Let me be clear that she didn't forgive his harmful actions. She forgave him as a human being who made big mistakes. This distinction is crucial!

You can forgive the person without forgiving the action. My client understood that her father did terrible things. She forgave him as a human being while understanding that his actions were wrong.

She chose to forgive for her own healing, not for his sake. She didn't tell him that she'd forgiven him during hypnosis. But here's the interesting part. After she forgave, her life improved emotionally, physically, and in her relationship with him.

Coincidence? I don't think so. I've seen this happen too many times to believe in coincidence. Out of her forgiveness, she created something wonderful.

When you forgive, the other person no longer has power over you. When you forgive, you move beyond the past and live more in the present. Don't forgive for their sake; forgive because you care about yourself. Forgiveness also applies to oneself. If you did something wrong, forgive yourself. It releases positive energy that's been trapped inside.

2. Fear
Holding onto fear can be like holding onto a big snake. You struggle to control an animal that's desperately trying to get loose. Here are a few types of fear that may hinder healing.

Fear of failure
Mary had her hopes dashed too many times in life. She called in sick today, missing the management exam at work. Part of her wants the promotion, but part of her thinks that it's safer not to take risks, so she can avoid the pain of failure. Sadly, she remains unaware of her internal conflict.

She wonders why she gets sick on important days but chalks it up to coincidence. Her fear of failure leads to unhappiness, but her subconscious doesn't see it that way.

Fear of success
Janet has suffered from a chronic condition for years. She thinks, "What happens if I recover fully? Then what?"

Her subconscious fears what life would be like if she was healthy. That fear can hinder healing. It may not make sense to most people, but the subconscious doesn't follow regular logic; it has its own rules.

Fear of losing power
There's a classic story of an unpleasant woman ("Ms. Smith") who bullied her family, relatives, and friends through her illness. People had to be nice to her because of it. She ruled her kingdom.

The family doctor asked the family if he could do an experiment, and they agreed. He called the woman and said, "Ms. Smith, an experimental drug has been developed that can cure you! When would you like to come in?"

Well, Ms. Smith made an appointment but later had to reschedule; she made another appointment but had to reschedule. After a few rounds of rescheduling, the doctor concluded that Ms. Smith's power over her family (which she believes comes from sympathy over her condition) was too important to her, and she'd prefer illness to giving up power.

From a hypnotherapy perspective, I believe Ms. Smith is not at fault. Consciously, she certainly wants to recover. But subconsciously, she doesn't understand how to recover and keep her power, so her subconscious keeps her ill. In other words, if a person's subconscious hinders progress, it's often out of ignorance, not malice.

3. Self-worth

Heather is ill, and consciously, she says, "I want to heal quickly!" But during hypnosis, her subconscious says, "I don't deserve to get better. I deserve this illness. I'm a bad person."

If the conscious and subconscious disagree, often the subconscious wins. If her subconscious believes Heather doesn't deserve to get better, then her subconscious may do things to hinder the recovery.

4. Identifying with a loved one

There's the classic story about a young boy who practically worshipped his father and emulated him as much as possible.

His father was kind and decent; the boy became kind and decent. His father loved baseball; the boy loved baseball. His father treated his wife with respect; the boy treated women with respect.

His father developed a heart condition at age 30. The boy turned 30 and developed a heart condition. Coincidence? Perhaps not.

He loved his father so much that he even emulated his father's health! I'm not suggesting that he consciously emulated his father's heart condition; it was a subconscious decision.

How often does this happen? I don't know; all I can say is that it happens for some people, though it'd be tough to research.

Sometimes I wonder about genetics. Based on the scientific evidence that keeps piling up, it's clear to me that genetics plays a major role in some health conditions.

Yet I believe that sometimes we attribute health problems to genetics that may actually be partly due to the subconscious, such as the boy emulating his father at age 30 with the heart condition. On the positive side, this also means that we have more power over our bodies than we suspect.

By the way, after the boy developed the heart condition, he resolved his subconscious issue and resolved the heart condition.

CHAPTER REVIEW

"Is it dangerous to listen while driving?"
Yes. Use your script in a quiet place, with your eyes closed.

"When do I listen to my script? How often?"
Listen once a day at the same time each day, or connected to an existing routine.

"Can I aim for multiple goals, or should I stick to one?"
Have one goal in a script, and use one script.

"How do I speak as I record my script?"
Each stage has its guidelines on pace, volume, and emotion.

"What equipment do I need to record my script?"
Use a computer, digital recorder, or cassette recorder.

"Since I began practicing self-hypnosis, I've noticed good things happening to me. Is this a coincidence?"
It's normal. Consider it a ripple effect.

"What if I'm not healing quickly? Am I missing a step?"
This is a complex question. A complex issue may be hindering healing, or it may just be a matter of time.

- -

Next are a few concluding thoughts.

CONCLUSION

The mind and body both possess amazing abilities that aren't fully understood by modern science. And I'm excited about research happening today that gives more evidence about the connection between mind and body.

Affect the mind, and you can affect the body. Affect the body, and you can affect the mind.

I encourage you to let this book be just one step on your journey of healing and learning about hypnosis. For more resources, visit my site.

www.HealingAndHypnosis.com

Practice what you've learned from this book, and continue increasing your abilities.

Thank you for taking this book journey with me. If you're suffering from a health condition, may you heal faster than you ever expected and appreciate the good in your life. And if you're not suffering from a health condition, may you appreciate your good health and the good in your life.

To your good health,

William Song

"Aerodynamically, the bumble bee shouldn't be able to fly, but the bumble bee doesn't know it so it goes on flying anyway."

Mary Kay Ash
Founder of Mary Kay Cosmetics

BONUS HYPNOSIS SCRIPTS

You may notice that these bonus scripts include only the suggestions stage; just reuse the relaxation and awakening stages you saw earlier in chapter 11. Feel free to modify these scripts to your situation.

Note on using these scripts
Don't say the words in brackets out loud; they're brief descriptions so you can follow the flow of the script or it's an instruction, such as saying when to pause.

Some scripts may sound like discussions; some have strange or awkward sentences. You'll see that there are many ways to write a script. Here are the topics of the bonus scripts.

- Allergies (Breathe Freely)
- Chronic Pain (Feel Good Each Day)
- Clarity of Mind
- Healing in General
- Pre-Surgery and Post-Surgery (Heal Easily)
- Weight Management (Enjoy Your Food)

Caution!
Read the important health cautions in the introduction and chapter four. It could save your life!

If you're considering adapting these scripts to an issue that's life-threatening or serious, use extreme caution! Talk to your healthcare professionals (i.e., doctor, hypnotherapist, etc.) to ensure you're using hypnosis safely. Be careful!

For example, if you're allergic to peanuts, talk to your healthcare professionals and still carry an Epi-pen (device for those suffering from dangerous allergies; it saves lives).

ALLERGIES (BREATHE FREELY)

[Discuss immune system and allergy.]
Your immune system is a wonderful creation designed to protect you from harmful substances. An allergy is created when your immune system mistakenly believes a substance is harmful. In other words, your immune system is protecting you from something that's safe.

There was a man who was allergic to pollen from trees and flowers. It made his life more difficult, because he'd get a runny nose, itching, sneezing, etc. But then he learned and practiced hypnosis. He spoke to his immune system in hypnosis, and his immune system began understanding that trees and flowers were safe!

He learned that he could breathe naturally like everyone else and enjoy the beauty of the outdoors. After his immune system knew the truth, he enjoyed being outside with trees and flowers.

[Ask immune system to consider previous story.]
How did his immune system develop the mistaken belief long ago? Good question! Once his immune system realized that trees and flowers were safe, he felt safe. So I ask you, immune system, to consider this story. If you've been hanging onto a belief that's no longer useful, consider letting it go. An allergy is just a mistaken belief. That's all.

[Ask immune system to resolve the allergy.]
Perhaps there was a useful purpose behind the allergy long ago. But it's now time to have the truth come out; it's time to realize that it's time to let the allergy resolve itself.

It's time for the subconscious to communicate more clearly each day, and you'll feel happier and understood. And the conscious mind will feel happier, too. In fact, you both win!

Yes, in the past, the allergy may have served a purpose. But now it's time to serve that purpose in a healthier way. If you have something to say, then simply tell the conscious mind more directly instead of using the allergy as a message.

[Get the subconscious excited about making the change.]

As you resolve the allergy, your life becomes even more productive, more joyful, more wonderful, full of more happiness. And that's an amazing feeling to have each and every day! Sound like a miracle? It's yours as you both are willing to work as a team. The more you and the conscious mind work as a team, the better life is for both of you!

[Be an unstoppable team!]

As you both unite more and more each day, together you create an unstoppable team! As you set goals, together, you achieve your goals faster and faster than ever before. As you both achieve your goals, you set new, more outrageous goals, goals that were unimaginable in the past. Truly exciting goals!

And with true teamwork, you achieve those outrageous and exciting goals and even set new ones at an even higher level.

Your mind becomes more clear, more focused yet relaxed, and your life is truly the one you've always wanted. Remember, this is your life. Subconscious mind, it's now your time to shine. You deserve to shine! You've suffered in the past, and now it's time to claim your reward.

And part of your reward is to have greater health and vitality. And part of that is to feel more clear each day. Because the healthier you feel, the more you can truly live a happier life! And the more you can help others to do the same. It's time to let your true power shine into the world. It's your time to shine! It's your time to shine! It's your time to shine!

CHRONIC PAIN (FEEL GOOD EACH DAY)

[Start off with a suggestion of strength.]
Each day your body becomes stronger and more powerful. The old behavior of noticing pain becomes uninteresting and rather boring, like a below-average film you've seen many times.

[Transform pain into a different sensation.]
On the other hand, each day the old behavior transforms into a different sensation, a sensation that may feel differently each day. I'll mention two people that transformed their former painful feeling into a much healthier new sensation.

[Tell Warren's story.]
Warren used to have chronic pain, but after learning hypnosis he began transforming that old feeling into a warm and tingly sensation. His tingling was very mild, and after a few weeks, he barely noticed it. Once in a while he pushed his body a bit too much, and then he'd notice his tingling getting strong, which was just his body's way of signaling that Warren needed to pay attention to the body. And usually, Warren responded quickly to the message and rested.

[Tell Paula's story.]
The other person who used to have chronic pain was Paula. After learning hypnosis, she began transforming that old feeling into a slightly cool pulsing sensation, almost as if her body was experiencing a breath mint without actually eating a breath mint. After a few weeks, she hardly noticed the cool pulsing sensation. Like Warren, now and then she pushed her body a little too much, especially when she went dancing.

She just loves to dance! Anyhow, when she danced too long, she'd notice her cool pulsing sensation get stronger, and she would rest. She understood and respected that signal, though being human, once in a long while she'd push the envelope.

[Discuss warnings, including false messages.]
For both Warren and Paula, they understood that they had the power to transform the old feeling into a new sensation. If the body sends a signal of pain, it's usually because it wants to tell you something; it's like a warning. Sometimes the warning is important, and sometimes the warning is like a false car alarm, one that went off by accident.

Let me be clear: Warren and Paula did not shut down the body's warning signal. They can still get a warning, but the warning arrives in a more comfortable way, as a different sensation. And if the sensation gets strong, they understand that the body needs to rest. And they understand that it's important to work with their health professional to monitor their health, to make sure they're staying on a healthy track.

You may be wondering how you can do the same as Warren and Paula, and one way is to learn self-hypnosis, which you're doing right now. Each time you listen to this program, you are strengthening your hypnosis muscles, so to speak. And as your hypnosis muscles get stronger, this program becomes even more powerful for your subconscious.

And as this program becomes more powerful for your subconscious, it can reach your body each day, reminding it that it's wonderful to transform the old feeling into a new sensation that's still felt, yet more comfortable.

[Get the subconscious excited about the benefits.]
With this new sensation, you can walk longer, dance, and do other physical activities and still feel good! Having choices improves your life. Being able to do more doesn't mean you'll push yourself. You'll have the option to do more, and still be careful, too. Rome wasn't built in a day, and perhaps you'll improve your skills faster than you'd expected. You improve your skills daily, especially as you listen to this program.

And that gives you even more power to transform the old feeling into a new sensation, a sensation that is much more comfortable.

Each day you let go of the old feeling more easily, letting it transform into the new sensation. You embrace the new sensation, because you gain so much more comfort, ease of movement, and even a greater sense of grace. In a sense, you reclaim your life.

One way to speed up your healing process is to speak to your body throughout the day. Feel free to modify this example.

[Give conversation example.]
"Body, if you need more rest, I will give it to you. If you need healthy nutrition, I will give it to you. If you need quiet time alone, I will give it to you. If you need anything, I will give it to you.

"And I will give these things to you without you having to ask. But if I forget, gently remind me, and I'll get right back on track. And I do this for you, because you are me and I am you. You're the only body I have, and I understand how important you are. I need you to be healthy and strong, so we can both be out in the world doing what makes us happy. We're both in this together, and we're both one person."

By having conversations with your body, even brief ones that last a minute or so, you create a better relationship with your body. And as you do that, your body listens more to what you say. So speak to your body throughout the day! It will appreciate it, and you'll heal even faster. And that helps you more easily transform the old feeling into a new sensation.

CLARITY OF MIND

[Start off with a suggestion of clarity.]
Each day you improve your clarity of mind. In fact, just saying or hearing the phrase, "clarity of mind," out loud or silently, gives you improved clarity of mind. Why is clarity of mind so important? Clarity of mind helps you to enjoy your life so much more, including feeling comfortable with yourself and comfortable around others.

[Link old anxiety to someone else; time shifts are useful.]
As your clarity of mind grows stronger each day, you focus more on all of the blessings you have, and the old thoughts of anxiety seem like a distant life, lived by someone else.

[Create a positive chain reaction.]
Having clarity of mind leads to useful and positive thoughts. Useful and positive thoughts lead to effective action. Effective action leads to successful results. Successful results help you create an even better life. Successful means more than just financial success. Successful also means living life your way. Accepting and embracing who you are. Successful means loving yourself and others as deeply as you possibly can.

Creating the life you desire comes directly from clarity of mind. Therefore, you improve your clarity of mind each day by simply letting the phrase "clarity of mind" come into your thoughts throughout the day whenever you need that extra boost of clarity of mind.

[Shift time some more.]
Here's another reason you value clarity of mind: life is so much more enjoyable for people with clarity of mind. In the past, you experienced life with less clarity, and life felt hard. But now, each day you improve your clarity of mind. Therefore, each day you face the challenges in your life much more easily than you used to.

In the past, challenges that felt tough would look much easier to you today, because you now have much more clarity of mind. And having clarity of mind helps you to enjoy your life so much more, including having a good social life and better relationships with those you love.

[Imply that you have clarity of mind; notice the "yourself."]
People with clarity of mind, such as yourself, have the same number of challenges in life as anyone else. The difference is that you are able to face your challenges with a smile and positive outlook. And you overcome your challenges so much more easily and many times it's very enjoyable and very satisfying to overcome challenges.

After all, if you had no challenges, life would be boring. So you seek out new challenges, always striving to be the best you can be. And you look forward to new challenges with a feeling of confidence and excitement.

[Deepen suggestions with the countdown.]
I will count from 5 to 1. With each number counted, let everything you learned in this program go deeper and deeper into your subconscious, allowing what you have learned to become a part of who you are. **[Count slowly.]** 5, 4, 3, 2, 1.

HEALING IN GENERAL

[Plant seed that others have recovered completely. Also discuss what you're already doing.]
A number of people have recovered completely from [name the condition].

You have an excellent medical team helping you, and you're doing a lot to help yourself. You're eating healthy food, exercising to strengthen your body, and using hypnosis to accelerate your healing process.

[Acknowledge that there have been challenges.]
It may be true that some days are easier than others. Yet even on the challenging days, you are healing whether you realize it or have yet to notice your healing. Sometimes healing happens on a deeper level before it appears in the physical world.

[Discuss power of self-talk and visualization.]
As you've already learned, how we speak to ourselves each day affects healing. For example, there was a man who had chronic pain and said, "I wish I could stop the pain." Unfortunately for him, he didn't know hypnosis and didn't realize that the more he talked about pain, the more pain he felt. He gave the pain more energy, more power.

What could he have done instead? He could've said, "I focus on seeing myself as 100% healthy." If he focuses on what he wants, rather than what he doesn't want, then he'll likely recover much faster.

So take a few moments right now to focus on your 100% healthy self. Watch a mental movie of you as 100% healthy. See yourself on the movie screen moving, enjoying many activities, etc. See yourself really living life as 100% healthy.

And as you watch this movie, begin to really feel the joy and happiness of what you've accomplished. You've overcome the old condition, and in this movie you're really enjoying your life so much more fully! **[Pause for 20 seconds or so.]**

I realize that it may only seem like a movie in the beginning, but after watching this movie for a few days or weeks, you may find that it feels real!

And once you've reached that point, you may notice that you feel more optimism, more hope, and more confidence in your ability to heal completely.

That's what often happens to people who begin to feel the movie is real. And your body may begin to really absorb the movie, too!

That means your entire being begins to imagine that this movie is real! And as that happens more and more each day, you may notice that your healing pace accelerates!

And even when you're not doing a formal hypnosis session by yourself, you may find that you're focusing on the movie throughout the day. And that means you accelerate your healing even faster!

[Discuss importance of excitement.]
Remember, the subconscious mind helps make real what it keeps getting excited about. And every time you watch this movie, you get the subconscious more and more excited! Constant positive talking to yourself and constant watching of the movie both make a huge difference to your faster healing!

It's like reminding a child about how her birthday is coming up. Every time she's reminded of it, she gets excited about her party and her presents! So excite your subconscious mind several times a day, and build that momentum!

PRE-SURGERY AND POST-SURGERY (HEAL EASILY)

[Discuss pre-healing concept.]
Some people prepare for surgery by using a method called pre-healing. It's becoming increasingly popular and has already helped many people to recover more quickly. People report that they recover rapidly, with reduced pain medication, or even zero pain medication.

Their doctors are amazed at their excellent results. It's time for you to amaze yourself and your doctors by simply using this creative visualization program.

Listen to this program before surgery and after surgery. In other words, use this to help you pre-heal and to heal after surgery. For simplicity, I will only use the term healing from this point forward. But you, inner mind **[another way to say subconscious mind]**, understand what the body needs to hear and will adjust the language as needed. Take what you need from this program.

[Introduce the forest.]
You look around and see a beautiful forest with snow capped mountains in the distance. The sky is clear blue, the sun shines its warmth upon you, and a breeze cools your skin slightly. You feel the temperature is just right. Notice how green and peaceful the forest is. You smell the crisp clean air of the forest. You can hear the sounds of small animals.

You feel very grateful to be in such a wonderful forest. You notice a path, and you walk along this path. Feel the leaves underneath as you walk, listen to the sound of the leaves underneath as you walk, and smell the leaves underneath as you walk.

139

[Introduce the healing stream.]
As you continue to walk through the forest, up ahead you hear a stream. Listen to the peaceful sound of the stream. As you walk further, you see the stream and sense that this is a special healing stream of water. Look at the beauty of the light shining on the stream. See the sparkling of the light.

On a warm rock, you see a cloth. You sense that the cloth is for you, to help your healing. So you dip the warm cloth into the stream and place the cloth on any area that needs the healing. Ahhh, that area is now absorbing the healing water's energy. You feel warm and comfortable.

As you feel the cloth on your skin, listen to the rustle of animals, the wind in the trees, and the running of the stream. You feel at peace in the forest. You feel fortunate to use this stream for healing. You feel grateful to use this water to heal quickly. This stream strengthens your body. In fact, your quick recovery amazes you and those around you. This stream heals your body more quickly than anyone could imagine.

Now, using this healing water, you recover quickly, easily, and automatically. This water is incredible! Imagine your body as completely healed; really feel what that feels like; see what that looks like. Imagine yourself as 100% healed after the surgery. As I count from 5 to 1, let all that you have learned go deeper into your inner mind and into your body. **[Count slowly.]** 5, 4, 3, 2, 1.

[Introduce the polished rock for pain control.]
You continue to walk through the forest and see the face of a very polished rock. As you near this shining rock, you feel the warmth of the rock reflecting the rays of the sun. You sense that this rock is a special pain-control rock, helping you heal and feel comfortable as well.

You turn your body so the warmth is shining onto any area that needs to heal faster. It feels wonderful to feel the warmth and tingling. It means you are healing faster than you expected and doing so feeling good. In fact, each day you feel better and better, healing faster and faster, becoming more excited at being free again, more active. Imagine yourself feeling great, doing all the things you want to do, and having total recovery. Really feel how great your body feels as it heals so quickly.

And remember this important thought: if you feel any sensation in your body, it's a sign that you are healing quickly. Let that sensation become slightly warm and tingly. Let that sensation help speed up your healing. As I count from 5 to 1, let all that you have learned go deeper into your inner mind and into your body. **[Count slowly.]** 5, 4, 3, 2, 1.

[Introduce the forest's immune system expert.]
You now walk further into the forest. Up ahead you see a woman in the distance; as you get close, you sense this is a great healer, someone who understands the body in a deep way. As you get closer, this great healer says, "You have done much to help your body. Now, it is time to complete the healing process and magnify all that you've done."

She says, "In a moment, you will feel energy flow from this special tree branch to your body, helping to boost your immune system. You may feel a special tingly sensation, different from anything you've ever felt. It means your body is strengthening its immune system, helping you heal more quickly, magnifying all the other healing you just did. So go ahead and lie down on this soft forest clearing, and let your healing magnify."

After you lie down, the healer places the tree branch above your forehead, perhaps a few inches above or even higher, depending upon what feels more comfortable for you. You feel a slight tingling sensation on your forehead, and it relaxes you even more deeply.

She then slowly brings the branch across your face to your shoulder and chest area. Each area below the branch feels that same tingling energy. You realize that this energy magnifies all the healing that has already happened, helping you to accelerate the healing even faster. She seems to sense how high to hold the branch, so it's always comfortably above you.

She then moves the branch toward your stomach area and arms. And she continues to move the branch past your stomach toward your pelvic area, legs, and then to your feet, with the energy flowing easily to each area under the branch. After she finishes, she says, "Now, focus your mind on the areas that need the most assistance. Gently tell these areas to heal naturally and easily and quickly. Go ahead and speak." **[Pause 10 seconds.]**

[Deepen suggestions with the countdown.]
As you follow her suggestion and begin speaking to those areas, you feel the tingling getting stronger. This means your immune system grows stronger each day to help your body heal quickly. As I count from 5 to 1, let all that you have learned go deeper into your inner mind **[another way to say subconscious mind]** and into your body. **[Count slowly.]** 5, 4, 3, 2, 1.

WEIGHT MANAGEMENT (ENJOY YOUR FOOD)

[This gets straight to the point without an initial discussion.]
Here are three ways to replace the old habit of overeating with healthier habits, and still enjoy your food.

[Be more conscious of eating.]
Number one. Instead of eating as you used to, perhaps it's time to be more conscious of eating. Savor each bite of food. When you eat, take a moment to truly see your food, smell it, and then gently take a small bite. Let the flavor linger in your mouth, gently rolling the food around with your tongue.

Fully taste each small bite of food; let it play inside your mouth. Then swallow that one small bite of food before continuing your meal. Savoring each bite, fully seeing, smelling, and tasting, helps you appreciate the pleasure of eating. Ironically, by appreciating it more, you feel full more quickly. Why is that?

Sometimes people eat without appreciating each delicious bite of food, and that can lead to what's called unconscious eating. But you are getting more skilled at conscious eating, meaning eating on purpose.

[Breathe to enhance the meal.]
Number two. You can also breathe more at each meal to enhance your dining experience. Before you take that first bite, sit at the table and breathe deeply three times. Give thanks for the food you're about to receive in the way you'd like to give thanks.

Then between each bite, breathe deeply one to three times. Unusual? It sure is! But unusual beats normal if it accelerates your progress! By breathing deeply, you become more relaxed and more conscious of your food, and it tastes even better.

143

[Move as Nature intended.]

Number three. You can also move as Nature intended. Some call it exercise, but it's not about exercise. It's about moving as Nature intended. We were not designed to sit at a desk all day long. We were designed to move! Modern society doesn't encourage movement, so we need to make time to move our bodies.

[Reframe the issue to caring about the self.]

When you really think about it, it boils down to you caring about yourself. It's about you caring about yourself in a healthy, loving way, a bit more each day. It's about increasing your happiness bit by bit, by expressing how much you care about yourself.

And one way to express your love for yourself is to care for your body by moving your body each day. And as you move your body each day, you may find you appreciate and savor the food you have. And you may notice a smaller portion satisfies you more quickly.

Also, instead of taking the elevator to your floor, exit one floor early and walk the rest. After a while, get off two floors early, and so on. There are so many ways to build movement into your day. Plenty of articles suggest ways, or you can also think of your own ways. As you strengthen and take care of your body each day, your body will strengthen and take care of you. Again, as I said, it's not about exercise. It's really about you, caring about you.

[Create a plan.]

If you're not sure where to start, speak to your doctor or health professional to create a plan. By creating a plan, you can measure your progress. And measuring progress can help you motivate yourself. When it comes to weight management, keeping track of what you do can really inspire you to stay on track more easily.

By moving around each day, you express how much you care about you, and the better you'll feel inside. And the better you feel inside, the more you'll want to take care of your body. And the more you take care of your body, the easier it becomes to gently and more easily shed the excess pounds while still enjoying your food.

Bottom line: it's time to let your true power shine into the world. It's your time to shine. It's your time to shine. It's your time to shine. As you shed the excess pounds, you may notice other good things happening in your life, because when you improve one area of life, often there's a ripple effect, creating other improvements.

It's been noticed by many people, and though we can't fully explain it, you can certainly enjoy it! So go shine each day! You deserve it!

"There is only one way to happiness and that is to cease worrying about things which are beyond the power of our will."

Epictetus
Greek philosopher

GUIDE TO FURTHER READING

End Your Carpel Tunnel Pain Without Surgery, 2nd Edition
Kate Montgomery, N.D.
2004. Sports Touch. Boulder, CO.
The old edition (1998) helped me to heal from chronic pain.

Break Through Pain
Shinzen Young
2004. Sounds True, Inc. Boulder, CO.
I wish I'd had this book when I had chronic pain.

Beliefs: Pathways to Health & Well-Being
Robert Dilts, Tim Hallbom, and Suzi Smith
1990. Metamorphous Press. Portland, OR
If you have a health problem, read this book! It'll blow your mind, but in a good way.

Self-Hypnosis and Other Mind-Expanding Techniques
Charles Tebbetts
1987. Westwood Publishing Company, Inc. Glendale, CA.
One of my textbooks when I was in hypnotherapy school.

Creative Scripts for Hypnotherapy
Marlene E. Hunter, M.D.
1994. Brunner-Toutledge. New York, NY.
Has a good selection of hypnosis scripts.

Heart of the Mind
Connirae Andreas, Ph.D., and Steve Andreas, M.A.
1989. Real People Press. Moab, UT.
A classic in the NLP field. One of my favorite NLP books.

Introducing NLP
Joseph O'Connor and John Seymour
1995. Thorsons. London, England.
A great overview of NLP.

Unlimited Power
Anthony Robbins
1997 (first Fireside edition). Fireside. New York, NY.
There's a lot of power packed into this book!

Using Your Brain for a Change
Richard Bandler; edited by Connirae and Steve Andreas
1985. Real People Press. Moab, UT.
One of the first NLP books I read. Great book.

The New Psycho-Cybernetics (updated edition)
Maxwell Maltz, M.D., F.I.C.S.
2001. Prentice Hall Press. New York, NY.
Hypnosis under a different name and very powerful.

Reframing: Neuro-Linguistic Programming and the Transformation of Meaning
Richard Bandler and John Grinder; edited by Connirae and Steve Andreas
1982. Real People Press. Moab, UT.
A more advanced book.

The Rainbow Machine
Andrew T. Austin
2007. Real People Press. Boulder, CO.
Case studies from an outrageous hypnotherapist/NLP practitioner.

www.ingramcontent.com/pod-product-compliance
Lightning Source LLC
Chambersburg PA
CBHW021157010426
R18062100001B/R180621PG41931CBX00007B/9